PHANTOM OF THE NIGHT

PHANTOM OF THE NIGHT

Overcome sleep apnea syndrome and snoring—
win your hidden struggle
to breathe, sleep, and live.

T. Scott Johnson, M. D. and Jerry Halberstadt

Foreword by William C. Dement, M.D.
Chairman of the National Commission on Sleep Disorders Research
Introduction by Colin E. Sullivan, M.D.

NEW TECHNOLOGY PUBLISHING, INC.
ONSET

Phantom of the Night™

98 10 9 8 7 6 5 4 3

ISBN 1-882431-02-2 (Replaces ISBN 1-882431-00-6)

™ Trademarks of New Technology Publishing, Inc.

NEW TECHNOLOGY PUBLISHING, INC.™

Cambridge & Onset

All correspondence to:
6 West Boulevard, POB 1737
Onset, Massachusetts 02558-1737 USA
Telephone: 508-291-1111, 617-661-3851
FAX: 508-291-1704
Sales: 800-67-APNEA; FAX 800-45-APNEA
email: sales@newtechpub.com
Phantom Sleep Resources: www.newtechpub.com

To M. M. W. for her optimism—T.S.J.

To Elana and Ari— "Though we sow in sorrow, yet shall we reap in joy."—J.H.

If I say, "Sleep will comfort me,
I will lie down to ease my pain,"
then you terrify me with visions,
your nightmares choke me with horror,
and I wake up gasping for breath,
longing to be dead at last.

The Book of Job

Contents

x

x

x

Acknowledgments

New information now enables physicians to diagnose, treat, and enable recovery from sleep apnea syndrome. The dynamic process of scientific and medical progress does not end with the discovery of a new treatment. Indeed, that is but the beginning of change. The whole health care system needs to learn about these new concepts and procedures. Informed patients can take an active role in this process. Together we must overcome the barriers of lack of information, laws, and payment systems created prior to this new knowledge.

Dr. William Dement, chairman, and other members of the National Commission on Sleep Disorders Research renewed our sense of the urgent need for information and education about SAS for both patients and professionals. Information, encouragement, and advice came from other pioneers of sleep disorders science and medicine including Larry Findley, M.D., Meir Kryger, M.D, John Remmers, M.D., and Colin Sullivan, M.D., among many others. No less important were the responses of other people in the sleep community—scientists, doctors, nurses, therapists, technicians, psychologists, home care therapists, business people, caregivers, as well as patients and their families. The Association of Professional Sleep Societies offered courteous hospitality at their annual meetings.

The publication of this book has been supported by several companies in the sleep industry whose products or services are used in the diagnosis or treatment of sleep apnea syndrome. None of the companies supporting the development or distribution of this material expected to influence the content to favor their products or services, nor have the authors allowed commercial considerations to affect the book. We are grateful for the support and cooperation which has helped us to make the book more accurate and useful for the benefit of patients and other readers.

Apria Healthcare (formerly Homedco, Inc.) provided a grant to enable the publication of the first edition and helped to introduce the book to the professional sleep community at the 1992 Annual Meeting of the Association of Professional Sleep Societies in Phoenix.

EdenTec has been generous in support of the development of the book and Ed Schuck, Chair of the Board, has offered advice and encouragement throughout the research and writing.

Additional sponsoring companies and their representatives have provided information as well as generous support towards the development of this book. They include: Dave Gast, Product Marketing Manager, DeVilbiss; Dave Stephenson, Director of Marketing, Nicolet Instrument Corporation; and James Campbell, President, LifeCare.

We are grateful to the several companies which supplied and gave permission to use the product illustrations and information in Appendix D.

We also wish to thank the following individuals who have read and commented on the manuscript and provided useful information, advice, and assistance. Frank Adams, Stephen Amira, Ph.D., Susanna Bedell, M.D., Bud Blitzer, A. J. Block, M.D., Mark Estes, Daniel V. Draper, M.S., Bob Faircloth, Dr. Peter C. Farrell, Mike Ferragamo, Steve Grunin, Ari Halberstadt, David Halberstadt, Curt Hiller, Jose Hernandez, Henry L. Kettler, M.D., Michael Lawee, Peretz Lavie, Ph.D., Krysztof Lenk, Evelyn Luchs, Suzan E. Norman, Ph.D., Lucille Seger, Renee McCormick, Cheryl McGee, Ian McLeod, Phil McManus, Daniel Pinkwater, Arlene Prizant, Scott St. John, Lucy Seger, Menachem Student, Ph.D., Stephen Texin, Kenneth R. White, Gordie Wilson, Dolores G. Lorrie Wright, and Pat Zander. Mr. Bud Blitzer and the Gazette International Networking Institute kindly permitted us to use information from the *Directory of Sources for Ventilation Face Masks*. The three states or conditions—awake, quiet sleep, and dream sleep—pictured by J.A. Hobson and M. Steriade as part of their research survey has informed our presentation.

To the many others who prefer not to be named and to any we have inadvertently overlooked, our warm thanks.

The best way to express our gratitude and repay all the help we have received is to strive to make this knowledge available in the most accessible and useful form we can create—this book.

Foreword

William Dement, M.D., Ph.D.

This book brings a profound message of healing and hope to millions of people who suffer needlessly. Snoring and sleep apnea interfere with the normal processes of sleep—and sleep is essential to health and life. This book presents, accurately and clearly, paths to diagnosis and effective treatment of sleep apnea so that those whose sleep is disturbed can become aware of the problem and overcome it.

Men, women, and children are afflicted by sleep apnea, a disorder in which the throat muscles of the sleeper collapse, restricting the flow of breath. Sleep apnea syndrome robs these millions of the refreshing sleep they need to cope with the challenges of their waking lives. The sufferer tends to be a snorer, whose loud breathing is interrupted by a choking halt in breathing that lasts from 10 seconds to more than a minute. Breathing resumes with a snoring, choking noise. The interruptions in breathing reduce oxygen flow to the brain and can cause high blood pressure and irregularities in heart rhythm. In addition, these disruptions in sleep cause excessive sleepiness during waking hours. Recent research suggests that snoring even without sleep apnea syndrome may also disturb sleep significantly.

Sleepiness is a global epidemic, and sleep apnea syndrome is a major part of the threat to our nightly rest. One of the first signs of this sleep disorder is snoring—something that we find amusing, irritating, even a sign that a person is sleeping well. But the results can be tragic.

- Fatigue accounts for approximately 40 percent of commercial trucking accidents, claiming more than 4,100 lives and injuring more than 12,000 persons each year. Most of these injuries and deaths—from 70 to 80 percent—happen to people other than the truck drivers. Sleep apnea syndrome is a contributor to driver fatigue and crashes. The potential for lawsuits for wrongful death and injury is one result of the tragic, preventable impact of fatigue.

- Adult males over the age of 40 are especially vulnerable to developing sleep apnea syndrome—leading to high blood pressure, constant fatigue, the breakdown of marital and family ties, and a diminishing ability to succeed at work.

- Children who have sleeping problems may have more difficulty learning and be inattentive and irritable in the classroom. Many children suffer from undiagnosed sleep apnea syndrome.

- In one nursing home studied, more than one third of the patients were found to have sleep apnea syndrome—but none were being treated for this problem.
- As Chairman of the National Commission on Sleep Disorders, I have heard testimony from both men and women who have described the disintegration of families, the financial ruin of successful individuals, and death—caused by the lack of refreshing sleep because of sleep apnea syndrome.

The nature of the challenge—to identify and to treat the millions of people who have sleep apnea syndrome—is truly staggering. We need to involve the public and the entire medical profession and to develop new methods for screening, diagnosis, and treatment in order to bring restful sleep to these tired people.

Until every doctor asks patients, "How are you sleeping?" as part of every examination, sleep disorders will continue to be untreated. Very few doctors receive more than a cursory introduction to sleep medicine. We need to convince medical schools to introduce sleep disorders medicine into the curriculum. But we can't afford to wait for a new generation of doctors to be trained. Patients with sleep apnea need to receive diagnosis and treatment immediately and to do so they may need to take their health care into their own hands and actively educate their personal physician.

This book attempts to educate directly the people who suffer from sleep apnea syndrome (SAS) or those concerned for such sufferers. The advice here is addressed to you, the patient, who have the motivation and need to sleep well–the quality of your life depends on it.

This book teaches you how to recognize the disorder of sleep apnea syndrome (SAS), to gather information, and to work closely with your doctor, sleep specialists, sleep disorders centers, and other health-care providers. This book gives the patient the ability to raise questions with your family doctor. And that doctor, confronted with a new way of looking at sleep disorders, can discover the field of sleep-disorders medicine. Without necessarily becoming an expert, your family doctor can learn to become sensitive to sleep disorders, to ask about sleep and sleep-related symptoms, and to work with sleep-disorders experts and centers for referral and support. If you can learn what you need to do to sleep better and live better, then surely your doctor can learn with you. If you have SAS and work successfully with your doctor through diagnosis, treatment, and recovery, your doctor will be ready and able to help many more patients. You have a responsibility not for your health alone but perhaps also the health of many others.

Happily, effective treatments exist for this disabling disorder. This book accurately presents the fruits of research in sleep-disorders medicine on the treatment of sleep apnea syndrome. It is a clear, detailed, useful, and sympathetic guide for the patient. T. Scott Johnson, M.D., a pulmonologist, researcher, and clinician in the field of sleep disorders explains the scientific and medical information that a patient needs to become a fully informed partner in treatment. Jerry Halberstadt, before being treated, experienced years of frustration and failure because neither he nor his doctors identified his SAS. He shares his experiences in order to help other sufferers recognize the importance not only of receiving diagnosis and treatment but also of getting involved in the treatment process. The authors were aided by many others in the sleep disorders community, including Boyd Hayes, my former associate.

The challenge before us as health-care professionals and patients as well as members of society is to put this book's solutions to work. If you are not treated, you are endangering yourself and may be a risk to others as well. If you take charge of your own treatment, you will improve your life and the lives of those you care for, and you will be part of a much larger movement to wake up vast numbers of the sleepy victims of SAS. If you or someone you care about might have sleep apnea syndrome, please work with your health care professionals to get treatment. This book will help you take the initiative in receiving diagnosis and treatment for sleep apnea. Do this for yourself. And do it for the rest of us.

Stanford University
Palo Alto, California

Introduction

Colin E. Sullivan B.Sc.(Med.), M.B. B.S., Ph.D., F.R.A.C.P.

My own interests in sleep apnea extend back over many years. My 'conscious' knowledge of the disorder began in the early 1970s. At that time I worked with the late Professor David Read; he had become interested in sudden infant death syndrome (SIDS) and sleep apnea—interruptions in breathing during sleep—had been proposed as the mechanism of death. In 1975, when we studied our first adult patient with sleep apnea, clinicians thought it was a rare disorder. When David Read applied for a grant to study the problem, the reviewers rejected it because the "...disorder is so rare it is not worth studying." Later, I was fortunate to work in Toronto, Canada, with Professor Eliot Phillipson. We wanted to know how breathing was altered by sleep. In those years between 1976 and 1978 we participated in the growing awareness of how important the arousal responses are, protecting us in sleep. I clearly recollect helping Eliot Phillipson's Toronto group to do the first sleep study diagnosing sleep apnea.

I returned to Sydney in 1979 and I began to study and treat patients with sleep apnea. In that first year I saw only five patients with sleep apnea. Indeed, the patients only started to come following articles in the local news, television, and radio. Following any such publicity I would receive many calls and letters. At first I thought that I had found the entire number of patients with apnea in Sydney! I was totally wrong. The numbers coming simply rose exponentially. Of course we know now just how common the problem is—I think at least 15 percent of men over 40 years have the problem. I also now think that many more women than previously identified also have the problem; the difference is that they don't have the same range of symptoms. We now know snoring and sleep apnea are major factors in hypertension, heart disease, and stroke. Sleep apnea of the central type occurs commonly in heart failure and treating the apnea can greatly improve such patients.

The extent of the chronic disability caused by this disorder is astounding. A colleague in epidemiology, when told of the estimated numbers of those affected by sleep apnea, described it to me as a "public health disaster." Yet, in all those years from 1979, when I started to see patients, I confronted total resistance from the medical profession—from my own colleagues. Indeed, my interests in snoring and sleep apnea was a source of mirth and even contempt: "What, you actually research *snoring?*" This resistance was also seen at the level of the primary physician. Most family doctors didn't know about and were resistant to finding out about snoring and sleep apnea. Invariably it was the spouse who recognized the snoring, the apnea, and the sleepiness and who brought the sufferer to me. A common story from the spouse was that their own primary care physician, when consulted about the snoring, sleepy sufferer, would respond by saying, "So what, I do that!" I have many hundreds of referral letters from primary care physicians which simply say, "This lady wants you to see her husband because he *snores.*" The letters clearly show that the primary care physicians thought the referral unnecessary.

Of course, in 1979 we faced the dilemma that tracheostomy, an operation to bypass the part of the throat which is blocked in sleep apnea, was our only real treatment option. Our discovery of nasal continuous positive airway pressure (CPAP) changed this with the first test in June, 1980. Within a few years we had over 300 patients using nasal CPAP every night. In those years we made our own equipment. Once again, it was the sufferers who were the force leading to this therapy. Of the first five patients who were tested in 1980, one had a tracheostomy. (He went onto nasal CPAP in about 1983, and the tracheostomy was closed.) Another felt so good after his first night's sleep that he wanted to try the CPAP device at home. At that time there were no suitable masks; they were either too heavy, or more importantly could not maintain a seal for nasal CPAP. The first successful mask was made by using a set of large nasal tubes made of soft plastic and then running liquid silastic which solidified after a few minutes to form a very comfortable nose mask which provided a seal for many hours of sleep. The pressure source was a blower like a reversed vacuum cleaner.

Thus our first patient went home with such a device in February, 1981. At that time he was failing at work; his apnea caused sleepiness and compromised his ability to function. On treatment he went on to manage a very large corporation. After over 10 years of successful CPAP treatment he retired, still healthy. Those were years of productive work and positive personal life. Untreated, this man would have lost his work, career, and family—and perhaps his life. I see him regularly: he is fit and thin, but still has sleep apnea. He remains on CPAP. He has trialled many different masks and is now on our latest self-forming, self-sealing "bubble mask." He is my friend.

There is no doubt that nasal CPAP, a non-invasive, very safe therapy for sleep apnea, has revolutionized our understanding as well as the treatment of this common disorder. It has allowed us to trial therapy on patients for whom we would never have considered tracheostomy and in doing so it has brought into view the broad range of disability. For example, the Stanford team have now shown that even heavy snorers with partial obstruction have marked improvement in daytime function when treated with CPAP.

During these last 12 years of continuing research, we have constantly worked on masks and new systems. Next to my own office is our workshop; there would not be a week that passed that my technician, Jim Bruderer, and I would work on a different mask design. The latest "bubble mask" came out of those regular attempts to improve masks. Of course, in parallel with these developments has been the evolution of sophisticated air flow generators. We are currently developing an 'intelligent' CPAP which provides the pressure only when needed. These, and many other advances, will make the CPAP device very comfortable for the user.

The greatest pleasure I get out of this work is to see people's lives transformed.

I would like those of you who do have sleep apnea to know that the condition has touched me personally. I remember that when I was a medical student my mother was a snorer and stopped breathing and that my parents slept in separate rooms because of that. I also remember that she "nodded off" at night. In July 1967, I was awoken by the silence at 5:00AM. It was rare for me to awaken so early. I found her dead. I did not know then, but I know now that sleep apnea contributed to her death. She had hypothyroidism and most patients with that condition have sleep apnea. So the 'unconscious' reasons why I have worked in this area and have found a treatment which works are now apparent.

When I was asked to read *Phantom of the Night*, I was reluctant to do so because of my busy schedule. I run a large clinical and research program so that most of my reading time is occupied by manuscript preparation and scientific literature. However, when I began to read *Phantom of the Night*, I found it difficult to stop. Indeed, it reminded me of my own desire to write a book about sleep apnea for those who have the problem or who are affected by it. Jerry Halberstadt and Scott Johnson have produced a very special account of the problem of sleep apnea; the reason *Phantom of the Night* is so informative is that it is written jointly by a sufferer and a physician. It tells the real story of sleep apnea. It is not a stilted scientific report and it is not a 'lay' article, many of which have been written over the years. Instead, it explains the science of sleep disorders medicine for the patient. It demonstrates the crucial roles of the physician and the patient in treating snoring and sleep apnea and the wonderful impact of proper care, restoring the life of the patient.

I believe that the book should be read by every general practitioner (GP)—the primary care physician—so that they can hear about sleep apnea from the sufferers' perspective. It may thus help to advance medical education by helping to overcome the resistance of physicians to sleep disorders medicine which I encountered. I know that after you read this book you will understand what snoring and sleep apnea are about; I know that you will now also feel what it is about and identify with the sufferers and their families. Of course, the book is a must for everyone with sleep apnea and their families.

University of Sydney
Sydney, N.S.W., Australia

PHANTOM OF THE NIGHT

Chapter 1

Learning to breathe, sleep, and live

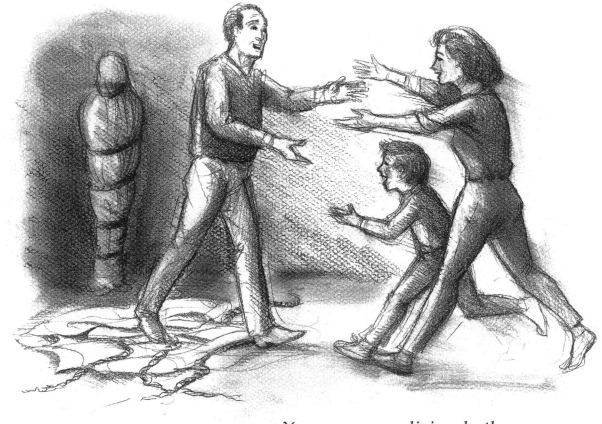

You can escape a living death.

Figure 1.1

Patient to patient

I am writing as a fellow sufferer and a patient to anyone who has sleep apnea syndrome (SAS). Every time I went to sleep, I snored and had pauses in my breathing. But I did not realize that many physical, intellectual, and emotional problems and my ever-present fatigue were related to how I slept. I wish that I could have read this book ten or twenty years ago, but nothing was available.

The purpose of writing this book is to provide you with information that can help you to return to a healthy, happy, and productive life. I hope to share with you information to enable you to assure your future. You may be one of uncounted millions of people with SAS who are trapped, as I was, in a half-asleep, half-alive underworld. This book provides information about treatments that sometimes seem miraculous in their effects. New advances in diagnosis and treatment could profoundly affect your life. As a patient, you can make better progress if you are well informed. Your experience, like mine and that of many others, may prove dramatic as you regain the wonderful ability to sleep well and thus live well. If you suffer from SAS, your problem may be more or less serious than mine. Fortunately, not everyone with SAS suffers the variety and depth of problems that I experienced. Certainly many with SAS suffer some degree of impairment, which may get worse unless it is recognized and treated.

People with SAS may find it hard to accept they have a problem, let alone deal with the idea that treatment may not be immediate and magical in every case. Although I met with many difficulties I believe that if I had been better informed, I could have overcome the problems and recovered faster.

More people, including doctors and other health professionals, are becoming aware of sleep disorders including SAS and offer us effective diagnostic and treatment alternatives. I recognize that some medical professionals don't want patients to hear about problems and difficulties in treatment for fear of discouraging someone from treatment. Nevertheless, I have described the impact on me and those close to me with the idea of sharing information and coping strategies. Much of this information may be useful to you only when you need a specific answer to your own situation.

My nightly struggle to sleep and breathe

Every night for at least 15 and probably for nearly 30 years, I was engaged in a life-and-death struggle. Two basic life forces were at war within me: the need to sleep and the need to breathe. This nightly struggle causes sleep apnea syndrome. Thus, sleep is a time of conflict rather than rest and recovery.

This exhausting struggle left me limping. I would awaken each morning not refreshed but like a battered warrior, ill prepared to face life's daily conflicts and challenges.

We must engage in another, daytime, struggle to regain health—to find the cause of our affliction and to obtain help. I learned that my adversary is called sleep apnea syndrome (SAS), or what I call "breath-less" sleep. I finally learned to wrestle with my adversary and have been blessed with the return of health and hope.

When I was having sleep problems, I never thought that anything was wrong with me. I felt that other people were unable to understand or appreciate me, and I could not understand why relationships never worked out. As the result of prolonged sleep deprivation, my behavior and responses had become abnormal; probably, subtle cues and behaviors had disturbed others or I was slow to respond. Later, when I was in treatment and feeling better, I understood what had been happening by seeing it happen to someone close to me who had been unhappy, lethargic, down, and depressed. My friend had been unsuccessful in his efforts to study or to find work. I could not find a way to motivate or help him. However, when his sleep disorder (not SAS) responded to treatment, he became a different person, easier to be around and with a lot more energy. I could see dramatic changes in his personality. And I realized that similar changes had come to me, changing me from a lethargic, depressed person back to my normal mode of enthusiasm and energy.

The path to recovery

My family life and business were casualties of my hidden sleep disorder. Doctors and psychiatrists on two continents failed to diagnose and treat my SAS. Finally, when SAS was suspected, it took two years of visits to sleep laboratories and doctors to get the treatment to work. When I began to get some relief—about one to three hours of treated sleep a night—I looked for ways to make the treatment more effective. I searched for a book about the subject but could find only one short article. I called the author of the article, T. Scott Johnson, M.D., a leader in sleep disorders medicine. I told him that I wished I had read that article years ago. I asked if he could recommend any books. He did not know of a suitable book to recommend. Within a few minutes, we decided to write a book for people with SAS. We wanted to make it possible for each person to get control of their treatment and their lives.

Dr. Johnson's wisdom as a physician shows in his desire to learn about the perceptions and needs of patients—if only every doctor listened so well. He recognizes that recovery and health are made up of more than medicine and technology. I have had the privilege of learning from Dr. Johnson the answers to the questions that an SAS patient might ask a doctor. He took me to lectures and meetings and introduced me to other leading researchers and experts. Using that knowledge, I have been able to cooperate more effectively with my own personal physician, doctor, sleep disorders physician, and other sleep specialists. Now, by working with my physician, other experts, and other patients, I have learned how to improve my treatment success. Although some problems remain, I average six to eight hours of sleep per night—and I feel good.

I am no longer exhausted, confused, irritable, and depressed. I look forward to each day; the days are not long enough to do everything that I want to do. For the first time in many years, I am able to use my mind and intellect fully. Shadowy barriers that impeded my every thought and move have fallen away. Difficult personal and business relationships have become more rewarding. I am experiencing a continual transformation to an improved outlook, increased energy, and excitement in being alive. It's like falling in love—every ordinary experience is invested with new beauty and meaning. I feel a youthful vigor and enthusiasm that I have not known for many years. I am able to work much more efficiently as the treatment for my sleep apnea condition becomes more effective.

Treatment is a collaboration of many partners. In this book, Dr. Johnson and I have distilled the experience and knowledge won from research and treatment by many pioneering scientists, doctors, psychologists, therapists, nurses, technicians, and others in the healing professions as well as patients.

My wish for each of you who suffer from sleep apnea syndrome is that you will soon experience a full, speedy recovery and hear your spouse, friends, children, and associates exclaim about your miraculous return to health. And may it happen in ten days, not in ten months or ten years.—J.H.

You can do something about fatigue.

Being tired all the time is not normal or healthy, and may be dangerous—causing car accidents, for instance. You may be sleepy in the daytime for many reasons. Perhaps you are holding down two jobs or working a night shift. Maybe you just don't take the time to get the sleep you need. However, if you snore and experience daytime fatigue or you can't stop yourself from falling asleep during the day, you may be suffering from sleep apnea syndrome (SAS). This condition affects millions of people and is truly a phantom of the night–hidden from you while you sleep so you may never suspect it.

When you go to sleep, the muscles of the throat relax as a normal part of the sleep process. However, this relaxation may lead to a partial closure of the throat, causing a vibration that we hear as snoring. In individuals with SAS, this relaxation progresses to the point where the passage for air is blocked completely, which stops the breath. The brain responds by waking the patient up a little to open the air passage. Breathing begins again, but the natural sleep cycle is interrupted. *Sleep apnea* refers to the disruption of sleep by a blockage of breathing; *apnea* means "without breath."

Benefits of treating sleep apnea

Sleep disorders may rob you of your capacity to enjoy life and keep you from your goals, no matter how hard you try. Treatment can help most people who have SAS. With successful treatment, you can:

- Add more years to your life and improve its quality.
- Feel alive, strong, more vigorous.
- Have the energy and drive to achieve what you set out to do each day.
- Wake up refreshed each morning.
- Wake up without a headache.
- Be more intelligent and competent.
- Have better relationships with those close to you.
- Be more successful in your work (or education).
- Be able to take better care of your family.
- Stop feeling depressed.
- Avoid a heart attack or stroke.
- Lose weight more easily.
- Have interest in and enjoy better sex.
- Have more enjoyment and fun in life.
- Be in control of your life.

To individuals with SAS

Focusing on the most common type of sleep apnea, called obstructive sleep apnea, this book provides information for people suffering from sleep apnea syndrome (SAS) and may also be useful to people with severe snoring, which may also disrupt sleep. Other, rarer types of sleep apnea will not be discussed. The book will give you the essential information you need to begin the journey to diagnosis and treatment. We encourage you to start or continue a dialogue with your family and doctor that could lead to your recovery and the realization of your potential. Together you can identify most causes of daytime sleepiness and perhaps achieve dramatic improvement.

To the spouse, child, friend, or colleague

You can play an important role in the recovery of your friend, loved one, or colleague by offering patience and support. Sleep disorders are insidious and hard to identify and may cause symptoms and problems that have no apparent connection to sleep. The information in this book can help you understand the medical, technical, emotional, social, and psychological issues confronting the sleep apnea patient, and enable you to contribute to his or her recovery.

A word of caution

Our mission is to help bridge the gap between scientific medicine and the people whose lives it could transform. The purpose of this book is to help you, the reader, work with your doctor to determine if you have sleep apnea syndrome, to obtain a diagnosis, and to seek treatment and rehabilitation using appropriate medical, professional, personal, family, and community resources.

While we encourage you, the patient, to be an informed and active consumer of medical services, nothing in this book is intended to replace medical advice. Only your doctor, working with you, can make professional medical decisions that are right for you. Perhaps the single message of this book is to encourage you to work with your doctor: Please don't attempt to diagnose or treat yourself alone. For additional information, please consult your physician and the associations and support groups listed in Appendix A on page 121.

A challenge for patients, doctors, and society

SAS—an urgent problem

Millions of working people in the United States are debilitated from the struggle to breathe during sleep. In the New England Journal of Medicine (April, 1993), Terry Young and others reported on a study of working, middle-aged Americans. Based on their research, the frequency of disturbed breathing during sleep has been estimated at 24 percent for men and nine percent for women while the frequency of clinically important sleep apnea is estimated at four percent for men and two percent for women. No wonder Dr. Eliot Phillipson, in an editorial which appeared in the same publication, has called sleep apnea "a major public health problem." There may be as many as 30 million snorers in the United States, about 12 percent of the population. Snoring may indicate the presence of SAS, and may itself disrupt sleep.

The problems caused by snoring and SAS can be treated. We believe that urgent efforts to identify and treat SAS sufferers, especially those who are severely affected, should be made. But the resources to treat so many people are not available. In the United States, there are over 250 accredited and an estimated 500 to 1,200 or more nonaccredited sleep laboratories, each capable of handling 200-300 patients a year. Even if all these laboratories were to devote their entire resources to the diagnosis and treatment of SAS, it would take 25 years to handle the backlog of untreated sufferers in the United States. If more of these sufferers were to seek treatment, the existing facilities would be overwhelmed. Yet most people who suffer from SAS aren't even aware of the name or nature of their problem, so they don't know how to seek treatment.

SAS in the national health care debate

Clearly, society needs to inform and educate sufferers while creating the capacity to treat them. Despite the large number of people suffering from sleep disorders, including sleep apnea syndrome and snoring, these problems are hardly mentioned in the national debate about health care costs and priorities in the United States. Here is a major health problem which, thanks to scientific and medical progress, can be readily treated. Yet society has not yet allocated the resources to educate the public to help identify and overcome it. Nor has society yet provided an adequate supply of trained people and institutions that would suffice for the diagnosis and treatment of SAS. A comprehensive program would include financing for public education, a treatment system, and continuing research and professional education. The costs of such a program would more than likely be small compared to the economic benefits for society as well as for the individual sufferer.

Figure 1.2   Snoring and sleep apnea in the population

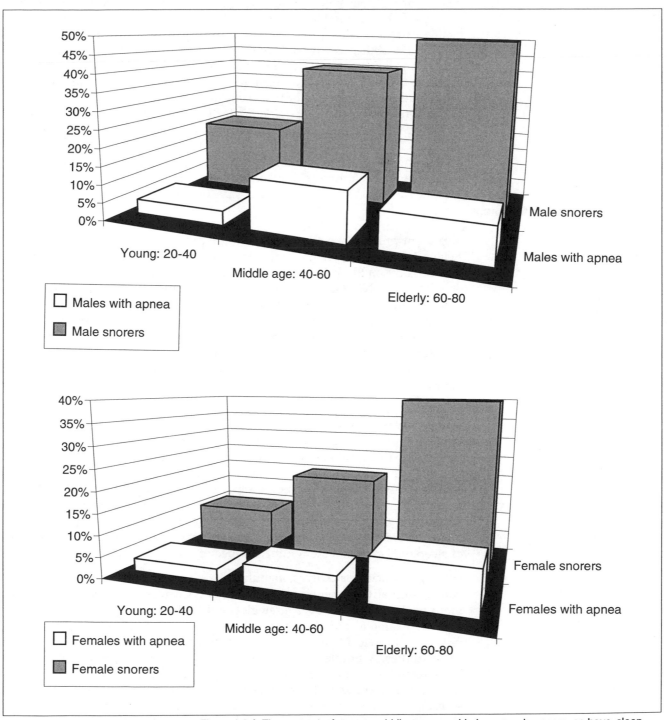

Figure 1.2.A The percent of young, middle-age, or elderly men who snore or have sleep apnea increases with age, except there are fewer elderly men who snore, compared to the middle age men who snore. Some scientists have raised the possibility that the decline in apnea frequency in elderly men may reflect the death of middle aged men due to sleep apnea.

Figure 1.2.B The estimated percent of young, middle-age, or elderly women who snore or have sleep apnea. Snoring and apnea increase with age in women, but the percentages are lower than in men of the same age. Some recent research suggests that the gap between men and women may be less than had been believed.

According to Daniel Callahan, a writer on medical ethics, we are faced with a health care system whose costs steadily rise. In his provocative book, *What Kind of Life*, he suggests that society must seek to balance the economic costs of health care with the goals and needs of both society and the individual. Because the ability to pay for health care is limited, Callahan sees the need to establish priorities and to allocate finite resources. He therefore proposes allocating available resources to treatable diseases where the patient will receive clear benefits. Currently available medical or surgical therapies to treat sleep apnea syndrome meet the criteria set forth by Callahan. Successfully treated patients can expect a longer life span, a marked improvement in cognition and ability to function, and the restoration of a healthy emotional outlook. Public education, identification of patients, and treatment for those severely affected by sleep apnea syndrome should be made a high national health care priority.

Strategies for the future

Important programs to educate health care professionals, the public, and physicians have been initiated. Following the recommendations of the National Commission on Sleep Disorders Research, a National Center on Sleep Disorders Research (NCSDR) has been created within the National Heart, Lung, and Blood Institute of the National Institutes of Health. The NCSDR will serve four key functions: to focus and coordinate a wide range of activities in sleep and sleep disorders, to support basic and clinical research, to train scientists, and to transfer technology to health professionals, policy makers, patients, and the public. A study of the cardiopulmonary consequences of sleep apnea is planned.

In another effort, William Dement has initiated a program—the Stanford University Sleep Disorders Awareness Project—that is designed to prepare the practicing physician and other health care professionals to identify, treat, and manage sleep apnea and other sleep disorders. This training program teaches practical procedures adapted to the routines of the primary care physician, enabling them to recognize the presence of sleep apnea and to manage treatment. Since primary care physicians have many patients under treatment for fatigue, high blood pressure, and other problems which may actually be related to sleep apnea syndrome, Dement hopes to disseminate the knowledge of sleep medicine into the routine practice of community medicine.

Clearly, physicians, scientists, manufacturers, and others need to develop innovative alternative strategies for diagnosis and treatment to cope with this enormous health problem. Such strategies could employ many techniques, including, for example, questionnaires which can be administered by the family physician to help identify SAS symptoms and the widespread use of home sleep studies. A simple test to identify sleep apnea is not yet in sight, but perhaps someday we may have a test of upper airway function that can be performed either in the doctor's office or at home. The next few years may bring smart treatment devices that can evaluate, prescribe, and treat the patient automatically. Some visionaries foresee and are working to develop devices that can combine continual monitoring with decision making to control the treatment process each night. Future devices would include monitoring functions which are today only available in the sleep laboratory or just beginning to be implemented in home monitoring. Such technological advances, coupled with public and professional education and innovative health care strategies, may bring relief to the millions who suffer from sleep apnea syndrome.

Chapter 2

Good sleep

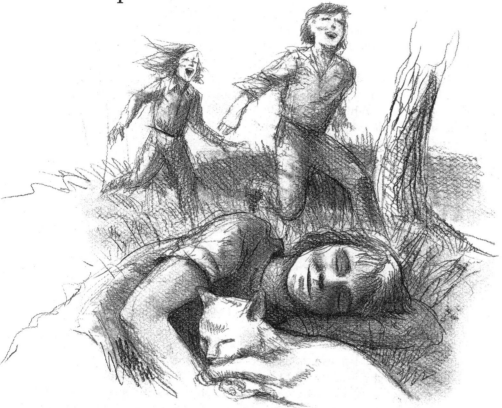

A child and pet animal asleep—so common, yet science is only now beginning to learn how sleep influences wakefulness.

Figure 2.1

What does sleep do for us?

We take sleep for granted. A child, a pet, a person—each falls asleep and wakes up as a natural event. Good sleep is necessary to be alert and awake. Good sleep means getting enough sleep at the right time to be fully rested and alert the next day. While we take sleep for granted, many of us abuse ourselves by trying to get by with less sleep. Our culture praises the worker who succeeds on four hours of sleep; it judges harshly a tired person, who is seen as lazy, immoral, and unproductive. Yet in people who have sleep problems something beyond awareness or direct control may impair good sleep. When sleep is disturbed we may not recognize what is wrong or know how to correct it. Since sleep apnea syndrome disturbs good sleep, it is useful to understand good sleep and why it is so important to sleep well, to better understand how to recover the ability to sleep.

Sleep and wakefulness

Dr. William Dement, a pioneer of modern sleep science, is often asked, "What is the function of sleep? What does sleep do for us? Why do we need to sleep?" Like a Zen master, he responds with the question, "What is the function of waking?" Every person's life is made up of alternating awake and asleep–two parts of an inseparable whole. Many experts in sleep use the yinyang symbol to picture the inseparable connection between parts of the fundamental rhythms of life: night and day, light and dark, awake and asleep. Each element is an inseparable partner in one whole. We think our lives as happening while we are awake, yet we can't be awake unless we sleep.

It seems obvious that wakefulness is necessary as a basis for survival. Behaviors and activities that we associate with staying alive are confined to the waking hours: earning a living, eating and drinking, procreation, the defense of our lives and property, teaching our children, or playing. Sleep, on the other hand, seems like a time of inactivity, vulnerability, a void or absence punctuated by the strange reality of dreams, a passive and vulnerable time that doesn't reveal its worth in obvious ways. But sleep is equally vital to our survival. Without sleep we are not able to function well while we are awake.

Daily cycles of activity and inactivity affect sleep and wakefulness

Everything alive has daily times for both activity and inactivity. Each day, plants open their leaves and flowers to follow the sun, then close at night. Every living thing is sensitive to light and dark and to changes in temperature. Each day the rising and setting of the sun act as timekeepers, while providing energy as light and warmth to enable the processes of life. In complex, advanced forms of life, such as primates and humans, sleep is the behavior that corresponds to the inactivity of lower beings. Just as plants and bacteria respond to the sun, so people have an internal clock that is set by exposure to sunlight each day. This internal clock rules the fundamental processes of the body, including when we feel sleepy and when we feel alert, when we are active and when we rest. This clock is our *circadian pacemaker*—it regulates a cycle of about 24 hours and sets the pace for many other events and processes. This clock is such a firm ruler that we can feel well only if we sleep at times determined by it. Thus people who travel may experience jet lag because their internal clocks don't match with local sun time. Their bodies and minds are trying to sleep while everyone else is awake, and they feel alert and active while local people are sleeping. People who work on shifts may have similar problems because their internal clocks are telling them to sleep while they are trying to work.

The daily need for sleep

Our days are thus made up of a routine: awake for approximately 16 hours, followed by about eight hours of sleep that include two hours of dream sleep and six hours of quiet sleep. Individual variations in the need for sleep occur—some people require more, some less than the average eight hours. If you have gotten your required number of hours of good sleep (including getting sleep at the right time, determined by the internal circadian clock), you wake up refreshed and alert. When you arise from sleep, another internal process starts running and determines the strength of your need for sleep. This process is like an hourglass that takes sixteen hours to empty—when it runs out, you will need to go to sleep again. If this pattern or sequence is disrupted, the normal balance of sleep and waking will be disturbed. If you haven't had your required hours of good sleep, you will be ready to fall asleep even during the day. Your internal clocks will put you to sleep unless you fight their effects with stimulants, physical activity, or extreme concentration. But even the slightest relaxation will allow sleep to overcome you.

Even patients who are haunted by the phantom of sleep apnea syndrome get some sleep every night (and during the day, even when sleeping may be dangerous or inappropriate). The drive for sleep is so strong that no matter how much it is suppressed it will ultimately take over. Someone who is deprived of good sleep is vulnerable to falling asleep at any time and can have many physical and emotional symptoms caused by fatigue.

The need to sleep is powerful. We have to sleep—as anyone knows who has tried to stay awake when very tired. Sleep will eventually overcome our desire to remain active and awake. One measure of the biological importance of sleep is its consistency throughout the animal world. All warm-blooded animals sleep; fish and reptiles also exhibit sleep-like behavior. Some animals can sleep while standing (such as cows) or perching (birds), and some actually sleep using only one-half of their brain at a time (dolphins and other sea mammals), while the other half of the brain keeps watch.

The three states of being

There are three conditions of our lives: awake, quiet sleep, and dream sleep. (See page 14). In each of these states or conditions, a different relationship exists between what a person's body is doing and what he or she thinks and feels. While *awake,* we have a reasonably accurate perception of what we are doing and we are usually active. In *quiet sleep,* we are relatively relaxed, passive, and lying down, and may think and even dream. Our thoughts and dreams in quiet sleep are a blurred, colorless continuation of our daily waking experience. In true *dream sleep,* the motor activity of the body is paralyzed. Our eyes may move quickly so dream sleep is called *rapid eye movement* (REM) sleep. Although we are unable to move, we perceive and experience vivid, sometimes seemingly illogical, impossible, and fantastic dream events. We fly, have conversations with dead or distant loved ones, flee from or vanquish horrible monsters, or recognize the disguised solutions to our daytime challenges. The experiences of our dreams seem to occur in dimensions and following rules of time, space, emotions, logic, and causality which are dramatically different from our normal waking state.

A trained observer can see and hear clues that distinguish which of the three conditions of waking, quiet sleep, and dream sleep that a person is experiencing. Even the untrained observer has little difficulty separating waking from sleep. For example, when a parent enters a child's room, he or she can tell almost immediately if the child is asleep. If the child is pretending to sleep with closed eyes, that is usually apparent. How can the parent so easily tell if

Figure 2.2 The three states of being: awake, quiet sleep, and dream sleep

| Awake | Quiet Sleep | Dream Sleep |

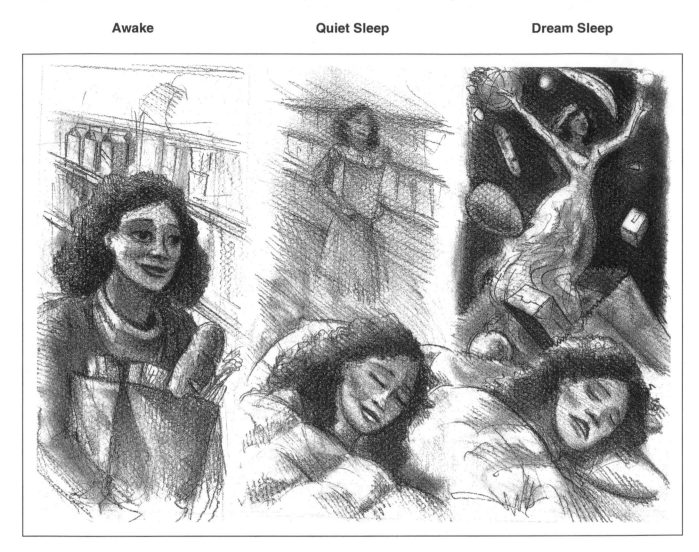

Figure 2.2.A **Awake** The external world dominates the reality that we live in. We perceive and respond to what is happening around us.

Figure 2.2.B **Quiet sleep** We shut out the outside world and live in calm quiet repose. The mind is uncluttered with only vague (but logical, realistic) thoughts present.

Figure 2.2.C **Dream sleep** Vivid, illogical or seemingly unrealistic fantasies generated by the brain become our dream reality. Our physical body is restrained but our mind is unleashed.

the child is asleep? One clue is the sound of breathing. A sleeper breathes slowly and more deeply, often with a slight sighing quality to the breaths. The eyes are shut, not tightly as when squinting, but passively, because the muscles that keep the eye open are relaxed. The sleeper is quiet but not immobile—moving the limbs occasionally, and swallowing, smacking the lips, or, rarely, gritting the teeth. This state of sleep is termed quiet sleep.

Dream sleep

A closer and longer observation of a sleeping person will provide the viewer with a clearly different set of behaviors, a second kind of sleep that most of us have observed in household pets. The animal may be whimpering and its paws may twitch, while breathing is irregular, with rapid short breaths interspersed with long pauses. We conclude, "Rover is dreaming of chasing a rabbit." In humans, too, this state of sleep is associated strongly with dreams and is called *rapid eye movement (REM)* sleep because of frequent bursts of flitting eye movements. One reason we rarely witness REM sleep in other people is that dream sleep usually does not occur until after about 90 minutes of quiet sleep. Unless we suffer from insomnia, we will be asleep before our bed partner reaches dream sleep. In contrast, dream sleep in a dog can occur quite soon after the animal goes to sleep.

Breathing during sleep

During quiet sleep, breathing is very regular, with eight to 10 breaths per minute. The monotony of breathing, both in rate and depth, reinforces the impression of the sleeper's restful repose. During this state of sleep, breathing is regulated by the need to bring fresh air with oxygen into the body and to exhale waste gas (carbon dioxide). Since during quiet sleep the muscles and organs are resting and using energy at a constant rate, the rate of breathing does not change. In contrast, during dream sleep breathing is irregular and even chaotic. Deep breaths are interspersed with shallow in an irregular pattern. Breathing seems to be responding to the internal events of the brain (dreams) rather than to the amount of energy that the body is consuming. Thus breathing during dream sleep is similar to awake breathing. While we are awake, breathing responds to changing levels of activity as well as to our feelings. Dream sleep is paradoxical—the motor muscles are paralyzed yet the brain is extremely active, and breathing responds to imagined, not real, movement and activity.

The functions of sleep

Sleep deprivation

Much of what we can say about the benefit of sleep comes from experiments in which people or animals are deprived of sleep. Subjects can be totally or partially deprived of sleep, or they can be deprived of either quiet or dream sleep. Scientists look for the effects of sleep deprivation in diverse places: the functions of the mind (memory, intellect, etc.), the temperature of the body, hormones produced, the ability of muscles to exercise, etc.

One of the most famous examples of prolonged sleep deprivation in humans was the experience of a 17 year old, Randy Gardner, who voluntarily remained awake for eleven days (264 hours). An inquisitive and adventuresome person, he decided to embark on this period of sleeplessness as a science project. He tolerated sleep deprivation remarkably well and his experience challenged previous scientific opinion, which held that such lack of sleep would inevitably lead to cognitive, emotional, or physical breakdown. Dr. William Dement and his colleagues, who monitored this boy's waking vigil, made additional discoveries. They found that despite the lack of sleep, the young man was able to function normally if he was actively moving and exposed to novel experiences and stimulation. However, in the absence of movement and stimulation he was very drowsy and performed poorly. While it is remarkable how well he could perform with stimulation, it is also sobering to consider some of the problems that emerged which are so familiar in cases of sleep deprivation. Some of the effects of sleep deprivation which Gardner experienced included: visual illusions, inability to see clearly, daydreams, mood changes, some loss of physical coordination, irritability, memory lapses, difficulty concentrating, and other effects on speech, memory, and concentration. Even today scientists are not sure what are all the effects of long, partial sleep deprivation.

Complete sleep deprivation may have more serious consequences. Oliver Sacks relates in *Awakenings* that one-third of those individuals affected by the epidemic of sleeping sickness that swept the world in 1916-1917 died quickly. Others died within about two weeks, apparently because the sleep-control portions of their brains had been injured (by a type of encephalitis) and they could not sleep at all—a tragic demonstration that sleep is essential to life.

Small animals that are deprived of sleep die within about two weeks. At first, the animals tolerate sleep deprivation but require much more intake of food. Yet, they don't gain weight and begin to look malnourished, with scruffy fur and sores on their tails and feet. Finally, they have trouble maintaining their body temperatures and they die. Let there be no doubt—life without sleep is impossible.

Activities found only during sleep

Many events and processes happen only during sleep; if they are necessary to the functioning of the organism, then sleep may be necessary. Some of the extraordinary and mysterious changes taking place in our minds and bodies during sleep include:

- *Transformation from a "warm-blooded" to a "cold-blooded" existence.* During dream sleep, the biological processes that maintain our warm body temperature temporarily shuts down. Perhaps this is the chance for nature to stoke our furnaces.

- *Huge surges in hormones* such as prolactin (a hormone that controls milk production by females) and growth hormone (a hormone that regulates growth and metabolism).

- *A fall in blood pressure and heart rate during quiet sleep and wild swings in these rates during dreaming sleep.* This relaxation of blood pressure control during sleep may be important in keeping daytime blood pressure normal. Many sleep apnea patients suffer from high blood pressure.

- *Dreams and more dreams.* Each of us dreams every night, even though we don't always remember our dreams. Because all animals exhibit dreamlike sleep, scientists believe dreaming must somehow be important to survival. One theory, advanced by Jonathan Winson, a neuroscientist who studies memory, suggests that dreaming may be part of an important processing of experience and memories. Dreams may help us to evaluate the events of each day and create strategies for success.

What is the function of these peculiar changes in the human body? Speculations among scientists abound. But, as Dr. Dement suggests, the function of sleep is unquestionably the preservation of the individual if not the species— for without it we don't function well while awake—so we can't live well and may die as a result of accidents or illness related to fatigue.

Chapter 3

Life without sleep

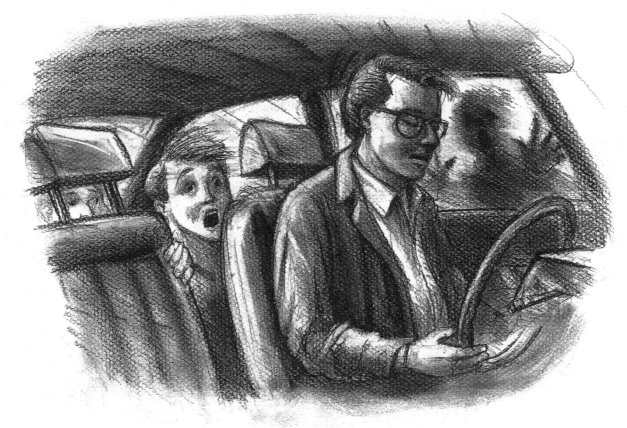

If the phantom has kept you from getting restful sleep, you can be so tired that nothing can keep you from falling asleep— possibly with tragic results.

Figure 3.1

My tired life

I fell asleep in buses, while watching TV, and even—briefly— while driving a couple of times. I had to take naps every day and was very aware of fighting sleep whenever I drove at night.

I was always exhausted, tired, and fatigued. It was hard to control myself—I was always ready to shout, sometimes even ready to hit someone. I was irritable, angry, and on occasion violent. I just wanted to be left alone, especially to nap. I was timid, almost paranoid. I found it hard to reach out to meet new people and explain my business to potential clients. I experienced a disturbing separation between my thoughts and feelings and my decisions and actions. It was as if two parts of my brain did not connect. It was hard to trust myself. I had pains in my joints, terrible headaches, and was depressed. Even today, if my treatment (for sleep apnea syndrome) has been uneven, I might feel tired enough to doze off.—JH

Do you have similar complaints?

If you fall asleep easily or can't stop yourself from falling asleep during the day or when you want to do something, you may have a serious sleep disorder that should be evaluated by your physician. If you have SAS, even though you sleep every night, you cannot get the restful sleep and rejuvenation necessary to function during the day. When you don't get proper sleep over a long period of time, many bad things happen. Your mind may be too clouded to interpret the danger signs correctly and you may lack the energy to respond to your condition.

Results of sleep loss

- You are always tired and have no drive.
- You get depressed.
- You are confused.
- You get angry and irritable, even violent.
- You fall asleep while watching your child's school play, operating a nuclear reactor, driving a truck, riding a bus.
- You don't do your job well; you can't concentrate; you're not productive.
- You think crazy thoughts, and at night you are visited by demonic dreams and feelings, or wake up over and over again.
- You worry because you can't understand why things go wrong, why you forget things, how you got from one place to another.
- You gain weight.
- You get in trouble with the law.
- You wake up feeling horrible and sometimes with a deep, awful headache.
- Everyone you know—even your spouse and family—is frustrated and angry with you.
- You may no longer be interested in sex or be able to have adequate or enjoyable sex.
- Nothing ever goes right for you.
- You deny that anything is wrong.

Any of these symptoms may have root causes other than a sleep disorder. Sleep deprivation can arise from numerous conditions or ailments. To determine if SAS (sleep apnea syndrome) is the source of these complaints, we must consider some more specific symptoms.

Questions to Identify sleep apnea syndrome

Answering the questions below will help you to understand whether sleep apnea is disturbing your sleep and disrupting your life.

The questions marked ♠ are especially important; a "yes" answer strongly suggests that sleep apnea is the problem. To answer questions marked with a ♥, you will need the help of your roommate, bedmate, or a family member, or you may use a tape recorder to identify snoring and pauses in breathing. For information on how to use a tape recorder, see Make a tape recording on page 110 in Chapter 10.

During sleep and in the bedroom

❏ *Do you snore loudly each night?* ♠♥

❏ *Do you have frequent pauses in breathing while you sleep (you stop breathing for ten seconds or longer)?* ♠♥

❏ Are you restless during sleep, tossing and turning from one side to another?♥

❏ Does your posture during sleep seem unusual—do you sleep sitting up or propped up by pillows?♥

❏ Do you have insomnia—waking up frequently and without a reason?

❏ Do you have to get up to urinate several times during the night?

❏ Have you wet your bed?

❏ Have you fallen from bed?

While awake

❏ Do you wake up in the morning tired and foggy, not ready to face the day?

❏ Do you have headaches in the morning? ♠

❏ Are you very sleepy during the day? ♠

❏ Do you fall asleep easily during the day? ♠

❏ Do you have difficulty concentrating, being productive, and completing tasks at work?

❏ Do you carry out routine tasks in a daze?

❏ Have you ever arrived home in your car but couldn't remember the trip from work?

Adjustment and emotional issues

❏ Are you having serious relationship problems at home, with friends and relatives, or at work?

❏ Are you afraid that you may be out of touch with the real world, unable to think clearly, losing your memory, or emotionally ill?

❏ Do your friends tell you that you're not like yourself?

❏ Are you depressed?

> ❑   Are you irritable and angry, especially first thing in the morning?

Medical, physical condition, and lifestyle

❑   Are you overweight?

❑   Do you have high blood pressure?

❑   Do you have pains in your bones and joints?

❑   Do you have trouble breathing through your nose?

❑   Do you often have a drink of alcohol before going to bed?

❑   If you are a man, is your collar size 17 inches (42 centimeters) or larger?

What your answers may mean

A "yes" answer to *any* of these questions may be a clue that an underlying disease exists. That disease may be sleep apnea, another sleep disorder, or a problem not related to sleep. Each of the questions points to a symptom. Symptoms are the clues, sometimes subtle and perceived only by the patient (such as memory loss), and sometimes overt and observable by friend or family (such as snoring) that indicate that the mind or body is diseased. Your doctor, trained to see symptoms as the manifestation of disease, can help you interpret and understand the basis of your condition.

Stories of other patients

A glimpse of these symptoms in other patients may help you understand the relevance of these symptoms to your sleep complaints.

You sleep when your life depends on staying alert.

Beginning at about age 35, Fred Hampton, an overweight man who drove for a living became increasingly tired during the day. He napped frequently at lunchtime. During trips he sometimes pulled off the road to rest when he became too tired to continue. His wife was aware that he snored, had interruptions in his breathing, and gasped for breath during sleep. No one suspected sleep apnea syndrome. At age 40, on the way home from work, within three miles of his home he fell asleep at the wheel and hit a tree. He suffered a spinal injury that left him paralyzed below the waist. Only then was he discovered to have severe obstructive sleep apnea.

The dangers of driving while tired

Sleepiness is a major contributor to 200,000 fatigue-related automobile and trucking accidents annually in the United States. Patients with sleep apnea have a higher risk of death than the normal population; automobile accidents may be one cause of this increased mortality rate. Although most people with sleep apnea have good driving records, the most severely affected one-third of sufferers of untreated sleep apnea usually have a bad crash record. It has been estimated that patients with untreated, severe sleep apnea have a two-to three-fold greater chance of having an automobile accident.

Unfortunately, many patients with SAS resist the idea of treatment, perhaps because they don't perceive or understand the effects of SAS on themselves and others. Often, a drastic event like a car crash finally shocks the patient or his family into seeking help for this sleep problem. According to Dr. Larry Findley, who has studied the effects of sleep apnea on driving safety, both the physician and the patient are responsible for the discovery and treatment of severe SAS because the untreated disorder threatens the well-being and safety of others, as well as the patient.

> The worst one-third of sleep apnea patients are usually very poor drivers who have an increased auto crash rate. These drivers may cause serious crashes and even fatalities. I have seen several patients who were seriously injured when they fell asleep while driving. These patients had untreated sleep apnea.

> I have seen air-traffic controllers, propane-gas truck drivers, bus drivers, and toxic-waste truck drivers with severe sleep apnea. Fortunately, these patients all received adequate treatment and became safe drivers (personal communication, L. Findley, M.D.).

You fall asleep while you work, listen to a lecture, or attend a movie.

Dr. William Farmington, a neurologist had been increasingly tired and was under pressure at work. Some patients complained because he even had gone to sleep while examining them. But he became aware of the extent of his daytime fatigue when he listened to a tape recording he had made of a lecture he attended at a conference. He was startled to discover that the loud snoring he heard on the tape was his own—he had fallen asleep during the talk. He received treatment for SAS and continued working in his demanding job.

If you are able to fall asleep easily and quickly during the day, this signals a problem, not something to be proud of. A healthy person who sleeps well can't fall asleep easily during the day, no matter how boring the circumstances. A person getting adequate sleep can't be put to sleep by a dull movie, a boring meeting, or an untalented performer. However, without sufficient good sleep you can hardly keep yourself from falling asleep, no matter how hard you try.

Being tired is a way of life.

Imagine how you would feel if you were awakened 200, 300, or 400 times each night. Patients with sleep apnea are tired and sleepy because of this disruption and fragmentation of their normal pattern of nighttime sleep. During the day they find it hard to stay awake to drive, read a newspaper, or carry out their jobs. Sleepiness may be irresistible, leading to serious car or work accidents. Yet getting more hours of sleep is not helpful, since the quality of sleep is poor.

You perform tasks automatically.

Especially while driving, John would snap out of a reverie and wonder how long he had been driving on autopilot. At times he would arrive at home from work and, turning off the car engine in his driveway, realize that he had no recollection of the drive home. Other times he would find himself turning into the driveway of his sister's house, who lived about five miles from him, when he had meant to drive home.

The ability to carry out a routine task in an altered state of mind is extraordinary—and frightening. Sleep deprived people find that they sometimes perform jobs such as driving from their home to work or to a friend's house without being aware of accomplishing a complex task. People might easily think they are losing their mind, but their minds are trying to snatch a bit of needed rest.

You (or others) think your personality has changed.

I was listless and only wanted to sleep. My wife and close friends—and even my doctor—thought I was suffering from depression.

I didn't feel like myself. And my friends told me I was different, not like my old self. What was happening to me?

He just wasn't the same person I married. People who worked for us in the store found it impossible to get along with him any more. He seemed to be looking for trouble.

Depression and other mood changes caused by lack of sleep

Changes in personality and intellect may be the only indication that a person suffers from sleep apnea. These changes can take many forms including irritability, sadness, or confusion.

Symptoms of depression and other changes in mood may result from sleep apnea syndrome. SAS is a medical disorder that may appear like a psychological problem or a psychiatric disease. Some of the symptoms seen in both sleep apnea syndrome patients and people suffering from depression include: fatigue, decreased task performance, low sexual drive, cognitive impairment, confusion, sleep disruption, lack of mental clarity, and low energy levels.

Treatment for depression with antidepressant medications may improve the mood of a patient with sleep apnea. But, if the underlying cause of the depression—disturbed breathing and sleep—is not recognized and treated as the source, treating for depression won't solve the sleep disorder problem. Although sleep apnea syndrome may create many psychological symptoms, SAS is definitely not caused by emotions or feelings. The symptoms of depression caused by SAS can be relieved by treatment of the underlying sleep apnea.

You have trouble maintaining stable and rewarding relationships.

I am having serious relationship problems at home, with my friends and relatives, and at work.

Patients with sleep apnea often suffer a breakdown in family relationships. Divorce is not uncommon. Potential sources of support such as family members or colleagues react negatively to the patient by withdrawing. The patient is too sleepy to participate in family activities without being irritable. Children are embarrassed by parents who fall asleep and snores at school plays, recitals, or other significant events. For many people, the loud snoring and persistent restlessness of their spouse makes sleeping in the same bedroom impossible.

You feel or act out of touch with the world.

I am afraid that I may be out of touch with the real world. Sometimes I feel unable to think clearly. I think I must be losing my memory, or maybe this is what it feels like to be mentally ill? I just don't feel like myself.

Some people suffering from sleep apnea may feel strangely disconnected from the world. This 'daze' represents the cumulative effect of the lack of refreshing sleep.

Figure 3.2   Out of touch

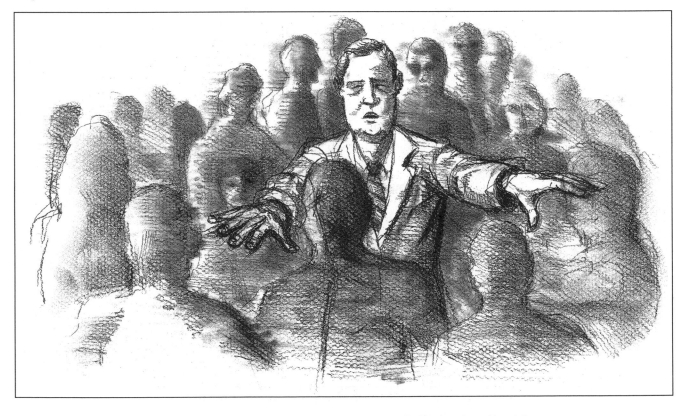

Figure 3.2   Fatigue can make a person feel and act 'out of touch.'

Preliminary evidence indicates that SAS may affect one's ability to conform to social constraints. A noted sleep researcher and clinician, Dr. Meir Kryger, M.D., told us that about one in 10 of his sleep apnea patients has had problems with the police.

You (or others) have noted problems with your sleep.

Snoring

I snore loudly almost every night. My wife tells me that she can hear my snoring downstairs. I didn't believe her until she used a tape recorder.

Snoring, especially loud nightly snoring, indicates that breathing is taking place through a narrow throat passage. For snorers, breathing during sleep is a struggle. Combined with other symptoms, especially daytime sleepiness, snoring demands medical evaluation. Even if breathing is not fully obstructed, snoring alone may disrupt sleep.

Apnea—interrupted breathing

I have pauses in my breathing during sleep. I stop breathing for almost a minute—at least that is what my wife tells me.

Loud nightly snoring (*habitual snoring*) may be caused by a narrow throat which is very relaxed during sleep. Such snoring is a hallmark of obstructive sleep apnea. In extreme cases, the narrow passage totally collapses, interrupting breathing, and suffocating the patient—this is sleep apnea. To breathe, the sleeper briefly awakens so that the air passage opens, and breathing continues but the patient pays a price in disturbed sleep.

Interruptions in breathing lasting from several seconds up to a minute are strong evidence that apneas are taking place. This symptom is one of the most reliable for determining if sleep apnea is a problem. The bed partner is usually acutely aware of these pauses.

When breathing stops, it is called *apnea.* This interruption in breathing is caused by the excessive relaxation of the throat. Snoring stops momentarily but instead of bringing relief to the tormented spouse, it brings anxiety about the next breath. Breathing usually resumes with a snort; often the patient will move or turn over in bed. This chaotic sleeping pattern can repeat itself hundreds of times each night.

Sleeping in unusual postures

They tell me I am restless during sleep. I awaken to find myself propped up on my arm. My shoulders ache in the morning from sleeping like that.

Patients may learn to sleep in an upright posture to maintain regular breathing.

Problems in sexual performance

Both my partner and I feel that my sexual performance isn't adequate.

Some men with sleep apnea are unable to achieve or maintain an erection. Although impotence has many causes, sleep apnea is one that can be readily treated, generally with good results.

Waking during the night

I wake up frequently for no reason.

Most people with sleep apnea are completely unaware of the hundreds of times that their sleep is disturbed during each night. Some, however, are aware of awakening fully several times per night. When they do, they may experience a sensation of suffocation or fright and a racing heart.

Urination

I wake up and have to urinate several times each night. I have wet my bed.

Normally, the circadian (daily) pattern of urine production shows a marked reduction in output during sleep. But people who suffer from SAS have high urine production during the night. However, treatment of the SAS reduces the production of urine to normal, low levels during sleep.

Falling out of bed

I have fallen out of bed.

Adults rarely fall out of bed. If you do, something is wrong, perhaps sleep apnea.

Overweight

I am overweight—but what has that got to do with feeling tired?

Obesity is a main risk factor for sleep apnea. Fat is deposited in and around the throat, narrowing it further. Snoring becomes worse, and finally total obstructions to breathing during sleep result. Often a small weight loss, even 10 to 15 pounds, can reverse sleep apnea and reduce snoring.

High blood pressure

My doctor has told me that I have high blood pressure.

Normally when we sleep our blood pressure falls. However, when your body must struggle to breathe all night because of sleep apnea, effort may cause the blood pressure to rise. During the day your blood pressure remains at a high level. In some clinics, about 30 percent of patients in treatment for high blood pressure are found to have SAS. With treatment for SAS, high blood pressure may be reduced, sometimes to the extent that blood pressure medication can be stopped.

Breathing problems

I have trouble breathing through my nose.

Any impediment to breathing freely through the nose can cause snoring or sleep apnea. A nose that was broken in an accident can impair breathing. Such maladies as hay fever, a deviated nasal septum, nasal polyps, or the common cold can be responsible. Nasal obstruction requires a stronger effort to breathe, which can collapse the breathing passage.

Joint pains

My knees hurt so much that I could hardly carry groceries, and the pains in my chest made me fear a heart attack.

Aches and pains may reflect the lack of restorative sleep. Complaints such as these may be found in other sleep disorders such as insomnia and nocturnal myoclonus, as well as in SAS.

Possible causes of SAS

Smoking

Yes, I smoke.

Cigarette smoking is especially dangerous for those whose breathing is impaired during sleep. Smoking irritates the sensitive tissues of the throat, narrows the breathing passage, and leads to excess production of mucus. Smoking also diminishes the ability of the blood to carry oxygen. Smoking increases the risk of stroke and heart attack; smoking and sleep apnea are a deadly combination.

Drinking alcohol

I usually have a drink (of alcohol) before I go to bed.

Alcohol consumption is especially dangerous for a patient with sleep apnea. A drink before bed—for relaxation or to promote sleep—may convert a mild snorer into a serious sleep apnea sufferer. Alcohol relaxes the breathing passage excessively.

Hope for SAS patients

Recognition of a sleep problem is the first and most important step. Once a diagnosis is made and treatment begins the patient can begin to put the shattered pieces of existence back together. When sleep apnea responds to treatment and the person begins to sleep well, mental and emotional recovery can occur rapidly. If SAS is recognized early, and if appropriate action is taken to keep it under control, the patient can avoid the tragic results that have affected untreated SAS victims in the past.

Chapter 4

Sleep breathing—a struggle for life

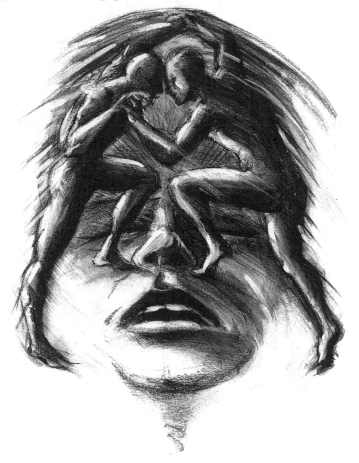

The internal nightly struggle between the two drives— to breathe and to sleep—causes sleep apnea syndrome.

Figure 4.1

Sleeping is not always restful

I had always believed that I slept well. I could fall asleep at any time of the day or night, so I felt I was something of an expert sleeper. I had no idea that instead of experiencing restorative sleep, I was struggling to breathe and to stay alive. Sleep was a time of conflict rather than rest and recovery.

Although I suspected that I had some kind of a sleep problem because of the pauses in my breathing and other symptoms, I didn't understand how my sleep breathing might affect my sleep and my life. For each of my problems and symptoms there was another explanation. Doctors and psychiatrists didn't recognize the possibility of a connection between sleep disorders and my symptoms. Nor were my physicians aware of an effective treatment for snoring or sleep apnea syndrome, although a new treatment had been discovered and demonstrated to be effective.

Even when I was finally in treatment for SAS, I didn't have a clear idea of what was wrong and what I could do to improve my health. Unfortunately, my doctors and sleep specialists didn't provide enough information and guidance. Until recently, I didn't know what a good night's sleep was, nor did I know what it felt like to be truly rested and awake during the day. —J.H.

Understanding the sleep apnea cycle

Each of us breathes continuously and sleeps about one-third of each day. Yet only recently have scientists begin to explore and understand how these two essential activities interact. Patients with SAS struggle to breathe and to sleep at the same time. This is a mortal struggle since life requires that these vital processes coexist. Life without breath is an immediate death. Life without sleep is a living form of death. In sleep apnea sufferers the body reluctantly chooses life without sleep.

Each time the patient with sleep apnea falls asleep and relaxes, the throat collapses and blocks the flow of air. Breathing is interrupted which awakens the sleeper. The person can't breathe while sleeping and can't sleep without breathing. This pattern of interrupted sleep—the *sleep apnea cycle*—interferes with the natural course of sleep and causes not only fatigue and sleepiness but many other symptoms and problems. *Sleep apnea syndrome (SAS)* refers to the sleep apnea cycle, its causes, and its effects on health. Sleep apnea may arise from more than one cause and it can lead to a variety of symptoms. Regardless of the underlying cause, the effects on the patient can be wide ranging.

Normal breathing

The talented upper airway

The key to understanding sleep apnea lies in the breathing passageway. Air flows into and out of our lungs through a winding series of air passages. The uppermost structures of this passageway are the nose, the mouth, and the throat, collectively referred to as the upper airway, shown in Figure 4.2 on page 29. The upper airway is used for breathing, speaking, and swallowing. To swallow, the upper airway must be able to contract and squeeze itself together to push food down toward our stomach. For speech it must form itself into a variety of shapes to create the many sounds of language. To accomplish these tasks the upper airway is made of flexible tissues and muscles. The muscles constantly adapt this amazing upper airway structure to each action: to swallow, to speak, or to breathe.

Figure 4.2 The upper airway

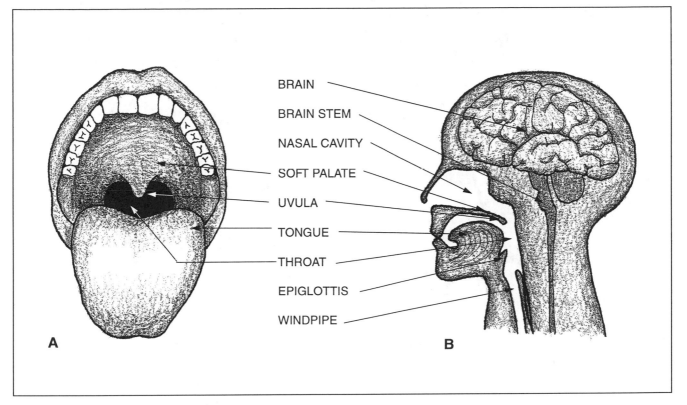

Figure 4.2.A The view of the open mouth shows the soft palate, uvula, tongue, and throat.

Figure 4.2.B The head and upper airway seen from the side shows in addition the nasal cavity, epiglottis, the windpipe or trachea, the brain, and brain stem.

To take a breath

This very flexibility, however, creates a problem for breathing, especially during sleep. To breathe in, air is drawn or sucked into the lungs from outside the body through this flexible tube (See Figure 4.3 on page 30). Air rushes through the nose, mouth, and throat as it progresses toward the lungs. This suction force tends to pull the flexible tissues of the upper airway together, narrowing and potentially obstructing this floppy passageway, much like a child can collapse a soda straw or juice box by suction. To prevent the upper airway from collapsing, many of the muscles of the throat must actively tense up to hold the throat open.

The coordination of muscle activity to maintain an open air passage for breathing is the responsibility of the brain centers (located in the brain stem) that con-

Figure 4.3   To take a breath

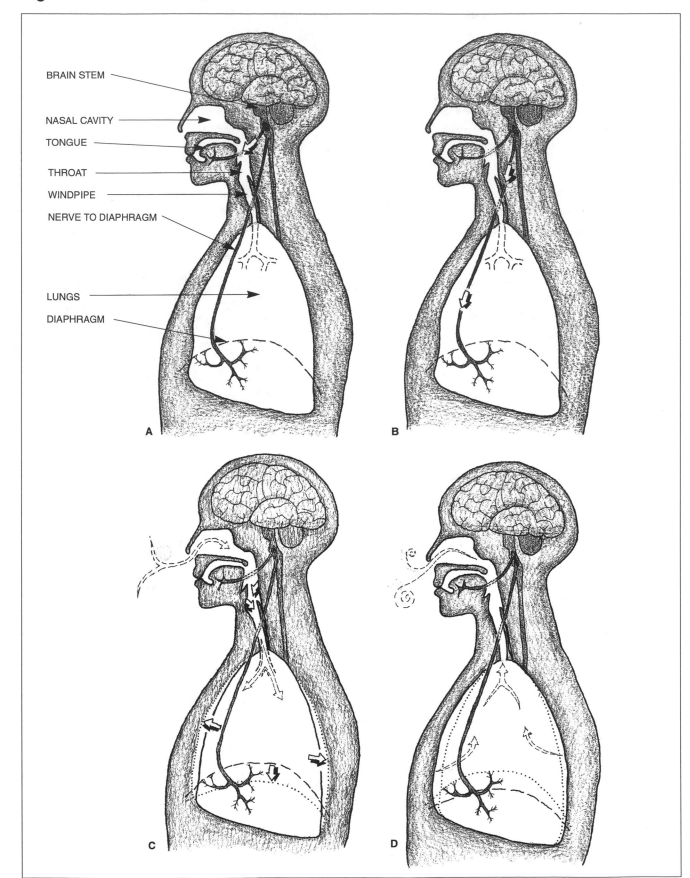

Figure 4.3   To take a breath

Figure 4.3.A Based on the time since the last breath and other sensory input, the brain determines when a breath is needed. It signals the tongue and upper airway muscles to become tense and thus create a rigid tube ready for the suction forces of the breath.

Figure 4.3.B Fractions of a second later, the brainstem sends a message by the phrenic nerve instructing the diaphragm to contract.

Figure 4.3.C Contraction of the diaphragm produces a suction force. Air is pulled into the lungs through the upper airway. Because the muscles of the upper airway were prepared for the breath, the suction force does not collapse the throat.

Figure 4.3.D When enough air has been breathed in, the brain turns off the signals to the diaphragm, chest muscles, and upper airways allowing these muscles to relax. Like a stretched rubber band that gets smaller when released, the lungs recoil and air is forced out of the lungs.

trol our breathing. Fractions of a second before a breath is taken the brain signals the muscles of the upper airway so that they have time to create tension, open the airway and withstand the suction force of the next breath. Then when the diaphragm (the main muscle of breathing) contracts and sucks in air, the throat remains open and allows the free passage of air.

Hiccuping is an example that shows what can happen when the muscles that open the upper airway are not coordinated with the diaphragm. A hiccup is the result of a quick contraction of the diaphragm without any signal to prepare the upper airway muscles. The rapid suction action quickly pulls together some parts of the throat leading to a "hic."

Breathing out is easy by contrast. Everything just relaxes and the lung springs back just like an elastic band that has been stretched. The force of the recoil of the lung and chest pushes the air out of our lungs through the upper airway to the outside atmosphere. Since the force is pushing air out of the lungs, the flexibility of the throat is not a liability—the pressure just pushes the throat open as the air escapes to the outside

Snoring

Snoring sounds come from a vibrating upper airway. In all of us the upper airway narrows when we lie down and sleep. This narrowing results from the relaxation of some of the muscles holding the upper airway open and from the pull of gravity on the flexible tissues, particularly the tongue. In some of us the narrowing progresses to the extent that the airway is partially blocked or obstructed. When a snoring sound comes from the throat during sleep it is an audible indication that the passageway has become too narrow to allow the free flow of air. There is partial obstruction. The floppy tissues vibrate as air is drawn past them, like a flag fluttering in a stiff breeze, creating the sound that we call snoring. The narrow place in the upper airway where snoring is most likely to arise is where the base of the tongue, the soft palate and uvula meet the back of the throat (See Figure 4.2.A on page 29).

The results of snoring

Snoring may be responsible for many ills. The noise alone creates a problem for anyone sleeping in the same bedroom, sometimes even in the same house. Many snorers also complain of the same symptoms that patients with sleep apnea have. This indicates that the noise or extra effort of breathing that

Figure 4.4   Upper airway relaxation causes snoring and sleep apnea

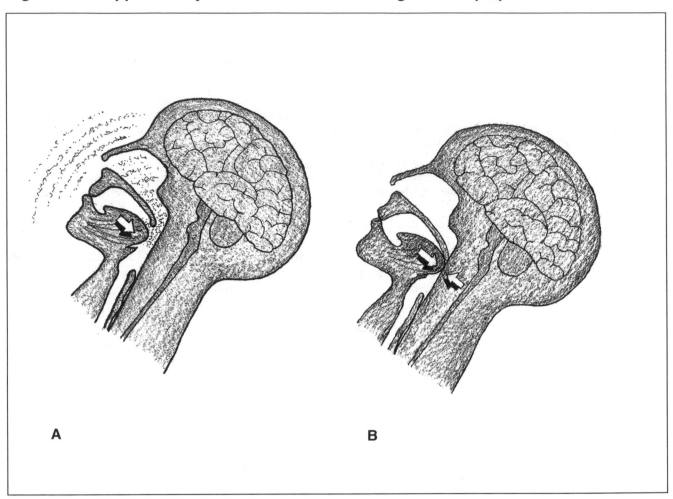

A

B

Figure 4.4.A *Snoring*. During sleep, the upper airway relaxes and the flow of air through a narrowed passage causes relaxed tissues to vibrate, generating snoring.

Figure 4.4.B *Apnea*. Further relaxation may lead to a complete stoppage of the airflow—obstructive apnea.

accompanies snoring may be fragmenting sleep just as apneas do. And the amount of trauma that the vibration of the tissues causes leaves them swollen and irritated. This is a vicious cycle because the swollen tissues cause more narrowing and obstruction and thus promote greater snoring. Fortunately, the adverse health effects of snoring have been recognized and snorers are benefitting from the knowledge gained in the study of sleep apnea.

Why do some people snore?

During sleep, everyone experiences some relaxation and narrowing of the upper airway or throat. But not everyone who sleeps snores. What factors may cause snoring?

A narrow floppy throat

A major difference between those who snore and those who don't is that snorers have a narrower upper airway passage even when awake. In a person with a narrow throat, the tissues that surround the opening are close together, which strengthens and speeds the flow of air past the narrowed area. There are many causes for a narrow throat, including obesity. Some people were just born with this problem. And for many patients we just don't know what the reasons are.

The muscles of the upper airway in snorers may also have less tension and thus are 'floppier' than normal during sleep. During sleep there is further relaxation of the muscles that control the air passageway. For reasons that are not yet understood, patients with SAS experience a greater loss of tension in these muscles during sleep than do normal individuals. This exaggerated relaxation coupled with a small narrow airway is responsible for the blockage during sleep. Yet during wakefulness the tone of these muscles is actually higher, probably related to the extra effort needed to keep open a smaller than normal airway.

Fat narrows the airway

Numerous surveys have demonstrated that obesity (being more than 20 percent overweight) is one of the most significant factors in the genesis of snoring. And it may be one of the most important since, unlike the facial structure that you were given at birth, being fat is something anyone can change. Why the association? It seems that the tissues that form and surround the upper airway readily accumulate extra body fat (forming double chins). This extra tissue narrows the throat restricting the free flow of air. When air is forced through a constriction in a tube, it speeds up and a greater suction is created, pulling against the walls of the tube—increasing the chances of snoring caused by the flow of air that vibrates floppy tissue. Many people with a large neck (for men, over 17 inches or 42 cm.) snore and have SAS.

A blocked nose disturbs sleep breathing

Some very important studies in otherwise normal men have shown that nasal obstruction from any source can induce apnea. Nasal obstruction comes in many forms. All of us experience the common cold from time to time. Others suffer allergies during the hay fever season, complaining of sneezing and nasal congestion. Some people actually have a growth (such as a polyp or a tumor) that partly blocks the nasal passage. A deviated septum can also limit the flow of air. Regardless of the cause, nasal obstruction promotes snoring. Because of the obstruction, more effort is required to draw air in through the nose. This extra effort shows up as greater suction pressure in the back of the throat. More suction pulls the tissues closer together so they are more likely to vibrate (snoring) or obstruct (apnea).

Alcohol relaxes the throat too much

Alcohol hinders breathing during sleep by causing excessive relaxation of muscles in the upper airway that should maintain the breathing passage during sleep. The association between snoring and alcohol consumption pervades the popular literature. The drunken sleeper is typically depicted as snoring. The wives of many middle aged men will testify to the disruptive snoring produced by "only a few beers." Alcohol also depresses the center in the brain stem responsible for the control of breathing—a special danger for sleep apnea patients.

Sleeping on the back can make matters worse

Lying flat on one's back (the supine position) impairs breathing. In this position the abdomen pushes upward and compresses the lungs. A large pot belly will cause even greater hindrance to free breathing. Equally important is the fact that the throat is narrowed when the sleeper is supine because the force of gravity pulls the tongue against the back of the throat. The upper airway may therefore become critically narrowed so that snoring and apnea occur. Some individuals find that turning to the side or stomach may alleviate this problem, but a sleeping person has no direct control over body position. Some find that elevating the head of the bed, sleeping on firm pillows, or sleeping in a sitting position (such as in a lounge chair) may help reduce snoring, but such methods usually do not alleviate the problem.

We don't have all the answers.

Scientists don't fully understand why some people are more likely to snore. For example, more men than women snore. Scientists aren't sure why this gender difference exists but it may have to do with the difference in hormones in men and women. After menopause, changes in hormones may explain why nearly as many women as men snore (Figure 1.2.A and Figure 1.2.B on page 9). Giving certain sex hormones to patients can cause snoring. As we get older, we are also more likely to snore. However, even children may have obstructed breathing (for information about children and adolescents, see *Solve Your Child's Sleep Problems* by Richard Ferber, M.D.)

Snoring is no laughing matter

Contrary to the popular view that the snoring sleeper is enjoying quality sleep, or that snoring is humorous, recent medical research shows that snoring itself interferes with the quality of sleep. Snorers breathe through an air passage that is narrower than normal. The extra effort required to breathe may also send a wake-up alarm signal to the sleeping brain.

The sleep apnea cycle

But even more ominous is the fact that snoring sometimes signals the presence of a potentially serious condition, SAS, which is certainly no subject for humor. Although both men and women of all ages can snore and have sleep apnea, we can say firmly that men have more apnea and snoring than women and that snoring is more common than apnea. The charts (Snoring and sleep apnea in the population on page 9 in Chapter 1) show estimated percentages derived from several population studies only to give a sense of the magnitude of the problem. While women seem less susceptible to both snoring and sleep apnea syndrome than men of the same age, some recent research suggests that the gap between men and women may be less than had been believed.

What is an apnea?

Snoring may progress to the point of complete obstruction of the upper airway. As sleep comes on, muscle tone in the patient with SAS slowly declines (Figure 4.6.B on page 39). Of particular importance is the relaxation of muscles that hold open the upper airway. These muscles have been working overtime during wakefulness to maintain the typically narrow passageway of the SAS patient open. Whether it is fatigue or some reflex action is not known, but with sleep onset the muscles relax enough to allow the upper airway to initially vibrate (snoring) and then obstruct (apnea). At a critical point, the tissues are flopped close together when the patient begins to take in a breath. The suction force of the air being drawn into the lungs through the upper airway is just too great and the airway is sucked close. This blocks the normal flow of air into the lung completely. This condition is called an *obstructive apnea*—the term *apnea* means "without breath." Since the body senses that something is wrong, each additional breath becomes stronger and stronger in an effort to overcome the obstruction. Unfortunately the increased effort only makes the problem worse by creating greater suction pressure in the already obstructed airway. By this time the struggle to breathe and the lack of fresh air flowing in and out of the lungs begins to disrupt sleep. An emergency message is sent to the brain about the problem with breathing.

The brain wakes up to start breathing

Fortunately the brain goes on alert. To end the apnea and get breathing started again, the brain 'wakes up' just enough to increase the nervous energy sent into the upper airway muscles. The tongue is pulled forward and other muscles contract, opening the airway, and several deep breaths are taken. This causes an explosive sound, like a whale surfacing, that spouses are keenly aware of. After the restoration of regular breathing, several refreshing breaths are taken and the alarm condition ends. The body is able to relax again and the aroused sleeper returns to sleep.

The sleep apnea cycle

Momentarily trouble resumes in the apnea patient. The relaxation that comes with the resumption of sleep closes the airway off again. The same chain of events is repeated, over and over again. This is termed the *sleep apnea cycle*. In a severely affected patient this cycle of sleep-obstruction-arousal can repeat itself hundreds of times in a single night. The internal struggle between the drives to breathe and to sleep continues throughout the night.

The loss of restorative sleep

This struggle to breathe may awaken the patient partly thus preventing deep relaxing sleep. Most often the person with SAS is unaware of these partial awakenings which are termed *micro-arousals.* But there is evidence that the brain becomes more alert and active during these periods. This cycle of events creates a disordered, chaotic pattern of brain activity completely unlike the usual progression of different kinds of sleep that marks normal, restorative sleep (see Chapter 6 for further details).

Rarely the apnea patient wakes up, gasping for air, heart pounding and head aching. The person who becomes aware of interrupted breathing during sleep can testify to its terror. Millions of others, unaware of their nightly struggle, believe that their sleep is normal and have no reason to consider that they may be awakening many times each night. Yet every night they experience perhaps hundreds of repetitions of the sleep apnea cycle: sleep, blockage of breath, awakening, sleep.

All snoring is not sleep apnea; all sleep apnea is not snoring

Although snoring and sleep apnea are often found together, the two are not always linked. There are occasional patients with obstructive sleep apnea who do not snore, or snore very little. Indeed, some patients who have undergone an operation on their throat can be completely freed of snoring but continue to experience apneas. In addition, there is a form of sleep apnea called central sleep apnea which is not caused by either obstruction in the throat or snoring. So, if you don't snore but do have symptoms of sleep apnea (like excessive daytime sleepiness) do not automatically conclude that you do not suffer from SAS or some other sleep disorder. Instead, discuss your concerns and symptoms with your personal physician.

Dangers of untreated SAS and snoring

SAS has serious consequences for health. It is probable that SAS carries more risk of early death—through cardiovascular disease, stroke, or auto accidents—than many other well known diseases that concern the public. Our knowledge of the health consequences of SAS is limited because researchers have only recently begun to explore the effects of sleep disorders.

Recent studies indicate that snorers who do not have sleep apnea may still have increased health problems. People who snore are more likely to have strokes, heart disease, and hypertension. This type of association does not prove that snoring causes these other conditions. Still it identifies the snorer as having an increased risk, much as an elevated cholesterol earmarks patients at risk for heart disease. In recent studies by Dr. Christian Guilleminault and colleagues, when snoring was treated both the observed quality of sleep and alertness on the next day improved immediately. Thus, there is reason to suspect that at least some snorers do not experience normal, restful sleep. People who snore would be wise to take steps to reduce snoring even if they don't have sleep apnea. Many of the suggested approaches to reduce SAS (See Chapter 9) also reduce snoring.

In addition to causing serious medical problems, the dangers of excessive fatigue caused by a sleep disorder extend to all aspects of life. Crashes caused by sleeping while driving is but one dramatic and tragic outcome. Since people with untreated SAS have intellectual, emotional, and physical changes which reduce their capabilities, they suffer indirect and direct consequences. These may include depression, poor performance in social and work settings, and the consequent failures and economic losses which can lead to the breakdown of family, social relations, the loss of employment, and unfortunate negative impacts on significant relationships.

Fixing the breathing problem restores sleep

One of the miracles of modern medicine is to enable a patient who has long suffered from the ravages of SAS to sleep normally by breaking the sleep apnea cycle. The treatment of choice—the one favored by physicians because it provides the most benefit at the lowest risk—is simple and dramatically effective, providing a good night's sleep for most patients, usually from the very first night. The method of treatment is to blow air through a mask into the nose under a slight pressure. The extra air pressure holds open the upper airway and keeps it from collapsing—it works like an internal brace or splint. Since air flow is maintained, the sleep apnea cycle does not begin and the sleeper is able to breathe and sleep at the same time. Fixing the breathing problem fixes most symptoms. This treatment method as well as the device used to supply air under pressure is called *CPAP—continuous positive airway pressure.*

Although sleep apnea was recognized in ancient times, effective treatment is new.

Dr. Meir Kryger has studied literary and historical sources and identified reports of probable sleep apnea as long ago as about 300 BCE. Dionysius, an extremely obese ruler, would fall asleep and stop breathing, so needles would be inserted into his skin to revive him. In 1822, William Wadd the Surgeon Extraordinary to the King of England, described the influence of obesity on breathing which was associated with daytime sleepiness. Charles Dickens, in the *Posthumous Papers of the Pickwick Club,* gave an extremely accurate description of a patient with sleep apnea—Joe, the sleepy messenger boy. William Osler, the father of modern internal medicine, referred to the connection between obesity and excessive daytime sleepiness in his influential textbook of medicine published in 1906.

In 1937 Annie Spitz, a physician in Germany, carefully recorded the sleep apnea syndrome. She commented on difficulties in breathing during sleep and noted that weight loss was an effective treatment. However, her observations were largely ignored by the medical community. Burwell and Robin used the term "Pickwickian syndrome" in 1956 to describe a poker player so tired that he fell asleep during a game—despite holding a full house. In a watershed paper, H. Gastaut described the cessation of breathing during sleep as the cause of symptoms in SAS. Dement, Guilleminault, and Kryger catalogued in detail the numerous signs and symptoms of the disorder during the latter half of the 1970s.

Tracheostomy was introduced as a lifesaving operation for sleep apnea in the 1970s. John Remmers made and reported in 1978 on elegant pressure measurements in the upper airways of sleeping subjects, contributing to our knowledge of the events in upper airway collapse. Colin Sullivan first applied nasal positive pressure or CPAP to treat sleep apnea patients, publishing his results in 1981. Since then, many scientists and clinicians have continued to seek the underlying causes and mechanisms of SAS in an effort to develop improved treatment methods.

Figure 4.5 The sleep apnea cycle

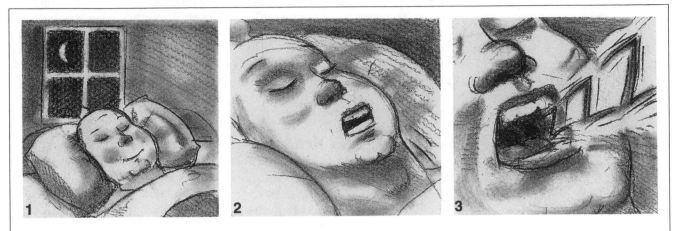

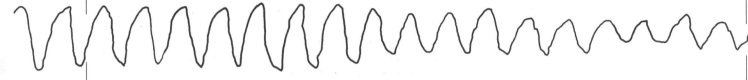

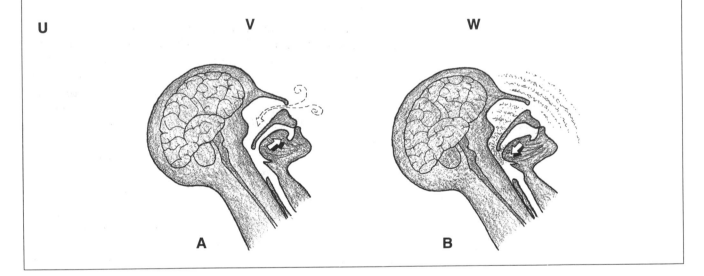

Figure 4.6.   *The sleep apnea cycle* is shown in drawings which depict what the unaided person could observe, in a simulated laboratory tracing of the respiration recorded at the nose, and in a cutaway series, showing the changes in the throat and brain. In the top row of drawings, a person is drowsy and falling asleep (1), falls asleep (2), snores (3), then becomes quiet as he stops breathing (4); he resumes breathing with an explosive gasp (5), and then, awakened, breathes quietly (6). The laboratory tracing represents the flow of air at the nose as the person breathes freely (U), then there is a reduction in airflow as the throat relaxes (V); the loose, relaxed tissue vibrates and causes snoring which further reduces the airflow (W); breathing stops as the throat collapses (X), then as the brain is aroused, the throat opens and air flows explosively (Y), there is exagerrated flow which then reduces (Z). Cutaway drawings (A-E) show the collapse of the throat and the arousal of the brain which account for these observations.

Figure 4.6.A *Sleep onset* Breathing is quiet and air flows easily through the upper airway, in and out of the lungs. The brain stem is sufficiently alert to maintain tension in the airway muscles, which keep the airway open.

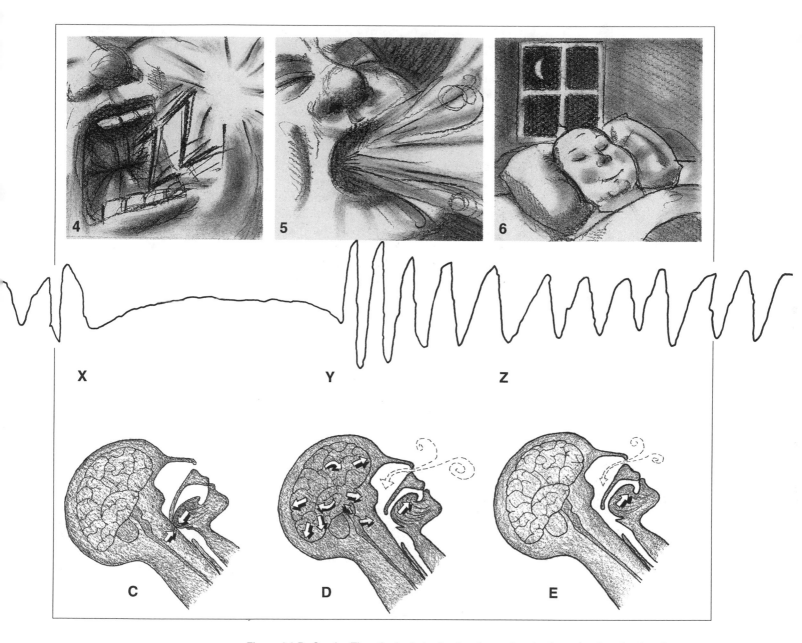

Figure 4.6.B *Snoring* Then the brain begins to relax and go to sleep. As sleep begins, the upper airway relaxes. Tissues begin to vibrate and the airway interferes with the flow of air to the lungs.

Figure 4.6.C *Obstruction* Further relaxation may lead to a complete stoppage of the airflow. Breathing is completely blocked by the collapse of the throat, creating an *apnea*. Therefore, neither breathing nor snoring is heard.

Figure 4.6.D *Arousal* The brain stem signals the muscles of the upper airway to open the airway. The arousal of the brain stem also arouses other parts of the brain, which disrupts the sleep process. Breathing begins with a gasp as the blockage is opened and then becomes quiet because there is no obstruction. But the ability to breathe comes at the expense of interrupted sleep.

Figure 4.6.E *Sleep onset* Again, breathing is quiet and air flows easily through the upper airway, in and out of the lungs. The brain stem is sufficiently alert to maintain tension in the airway muscles, which keep the airway open.

The application of positive pressure through the nose for the treatment of sleep apnea was a turning point in the management of SAS. Before that time, successful treatment was primarily limited to surgery (tracheostomy) that created an artificial breathing passage in the neck. Needless to say, this operation was performed on only the most severely ill patients. Nasal CPAP offers a safe, easy alternative for most patients with SAS and has become the treatment of choice. The advent and success of nasal CPAP has spurred interest in studying and treating SAS as well as other sleep disorders.

Despite the remarkable results which can be obtained using CPAP and other treatments, only a small number of the millions believed to suffer from SAS or snoring have been diagnosed and treated. Many doctors have not yet been exposed to sleep disorders medicine, nor is the public sufficiently aware of the dangers of sleep disorders. Education of the public and the professions is urgently needed. Perhaps the growing number of people who have enjoyed successful treatment for SAS will become teachers and advocates, helping others to recognize the symptoms of this common sleep disorder and urging and supporting these new patients to get effective treatment.

Chapter 5

Testing how you sleep

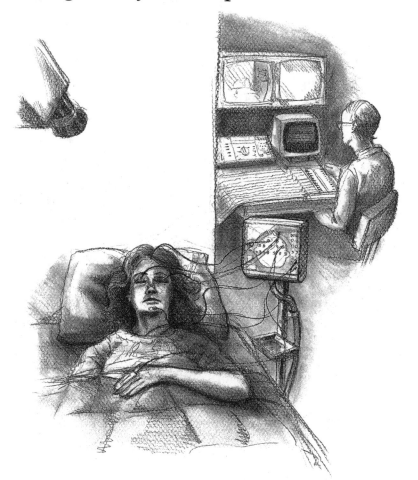

Testing sleep is a major step towards recovery. The way you breathe while you sleep may be the key that unlocks the puzzle and shows which treatment is appropriate.

Figure 5.1

Don't I sleep like everyone else?

Finally, a neurologist experienced with sleep disorders listened to my story and symptoms and concluded that I might have sleep apnea syndrome, SAS. When the first test time was available, I was ready for an overnight sleep test. Before the test I had to give up medication for two weeks. On the night of the laboratory tests

I was too tired to think. The technician attached many wires, belts, and gadgets to my head, face, chest, fingers, and legs, and offered to let me try on the mask that was part of the CPAP (continuous positive air pressure) treatment for SAS. I had no information about CPAP and didn't want to know about it. I was appalled at the idea of another awkward attachment and rejected the suggestion.

I woke up more than once in the night feeling strange, tired, and unhappy. The next day I remained in the hospital, with most of the wires attached. I was allowed to go to the cafeteria for meals. However, I had to return to the sleep laboratory at several scheduled times to take naps. Each time the wires were reattached to the monitor and I was allowed to lie down. I also had to have blood and urine samples taken.

When the results of the laboratory study came to my doctor, they showed clearly that I had "severe obstructive sleep apnea," or SAS. But I had to wait for another appointment for an overnight laboratory test to calibrate the correct pressure for CPAP treatment. More time passed until the results were available and I could begin treatment. The cycle, from tentative diagnosis to the beginning of treatment, took nine months.

Most people have an easier time than I did moving past the sleep laboratory experience to speedy treatment and recovery. I don't know why this qualified laboratory took so long. According to experts, my experiences are neither standard nor acceptable, although I have heard of other patients who had to wait a long time. Standards in competent laboratories are usually much better. The patient may have preliminary results in one to three days; treatment can often begin within a day or two, after one or two nights of laboratory work.

After treatment had begun, my doctor—a pulmonologist, or breathing specialist—suggested that a home study would provide useful information. I met with the laboratory technician, who gave me the small portable recording device. He explained and demonstrated how to attach the various sensors and turn on and verify the operation of the unit. At home I wired myself to the recorder, put on the treatment unit (see Chapter 7, The Miracle of Relief), which I was using on a regular basis, and slept. It was simple.

The next day, I brought the recorder back to the laboratory, where the results were read by the technician and doctor and reported to me in eleven days. The use of a home recorder meant that I worried less about delays in improving and fine-tuning my treatment. It relieved my concerns caused by occasional frustrations and mysterious failures to sleep well. Equally important, doing my home study improved my sense of control and competence. Now I work on a team with my doctor, laboratory technician, and others as a full participant in overcoming SAS.—J.H.

The science of sleep watching

During sleep, parts of the mind and body work together much as the instruments in an orchestra play together. If the instruments are not playing together, the orchestra doesn't sound right even to the ordinary listener. But it takes a trained musician to discover the problem by comparing what is being played to the musical score, the instructions. The musical score of sleep is based on the three states of being: awake, quiet sleep, and dream sleep (See The three states of being on page 13 in Chapter 2). Like a conductor who corrects the musicians in an orchestra, the person trained in sleep disorders looks for patterns that don't seem right and for their causes.

To solve some sleep problems, the best approach is to observe the sleeping patient. Although this idea seems new in modern medicine, in ancient Greek temples priests observed sleepers. However, since a sleep study today may involve attaching more than thirty wires to the body, sleeping in an unfamiliar bed, and having a video camera pointed at you all night, many patients are astonished that they can sleep at all in the sleep laboratory. Knowing what to expect before a sleep study should help allay anxieties and fears.

In the sleep laboratory, instruments record the 'score' of a sleep 'concert.' Each significant activity of the body is recorded separately and combined on a long piece of paper. Examining this night-long record can show which parts are working together and where harmony is lacking because of uncoordinated effort.

By studying the activity of the brain and eyes, and how tense or relaxed the muscles are, the patterns of being awake, in quiet sleep, or in dream sleep can be identified. Thus, different instruments record brain-wave activity, eye movement, and tension in the chin muscles.

Since problems in breathing can affect the quality of sleep, other instruments tell:

- if there is a flow of air into and out of the nose and/or mouth;
- if there is snoring, which indicates restricted air flow ;
- how much effort the diaphragm and chest are making to breathe, and if this effort is coordinated.

Since interruptions in breathing may affect heart rate and the amount of oxygen in the blood, other instruments record:

- the concentration of oxygen in the blood;
- the heart beat.

The information from these bodily activities and conditions, collected and printed on a long strip of paper, creates a chart called a *polysomnogram* (a written record of sleep). In a single night, over 1,000 pages can be generated. Some laboratories use a computer to record and analyze this massive amount of information.

This chapter and the following tell more than each patient may need or want to know about how these recordings are made and interpreted. However, you may find that this information will help you communicate better with your doctor. And you will find it useful to have a general idea of what to expect during the sleep study so that you can prepare for it and anticipate its potential benefits.

Preparing for the overnight study

Prepare for an overnight study by maintaining a regular sleep-wake schedule for several days before going to the laboratory. You don't want to be either excessively tired or alert from sleeping too much or too little for the several previous nights. In particular, a nap on the day of the study could make it hard to sleep that night. Since you will be sleeping in an unfamiliar environment, it is better to be somewhat tired. Most people with SAS are so tired that going to sleep won't be a problem. However, chronic fatigue may cause you to be sensitive, irritable, and impatient. Bring your toiletries and usual overnight items. A good book might help you fall asleep.

Another important issue is the continuation of medications, especially those that might influence sleep. Depending on the type of study and the type of medication you take, you might need to discontinue the drugs a week or two in advance. Check with your doctor or the laboratory about medications well in advance of your study. Pay special attention to nonprescription medications or alcohol because doctors may overlook their potential effects on sleep. If you usually take alcohol in the evening before sleeping, discuss this with your doctor.

In the sleep laboratory

Applying electrodes to the scalp

You will be prepared for the test by a technician who will attach test leads called *electrodes* to various parts of your head and body. Your head will be measured from front to back, side to side, and around, like a head band. The technician may mark your skin with a wax pencil to indicate the precise spots on your head where small metal cups with wires attached to them (electrodes) will be placed. These electrodes measure the brain waves that indicate if you are awake or asleep and tell which stage of sleep you are in. Since these signals are weak, they must be amplified, as a radio or television amplifies broadcast signals.

To capture a good signal from the weak brain electrical activity, the technician must ensure close contact between your scalp and the electrodes. The technician rubs a slightly abrasive paste at the site on your skin or scalp where the electrodes will be attached so the connection will be tighter. The signal captured by each pair of electrodes provides information, like that shown in Figure 5.2.A, that helps to understand and interpret the activity of the brain.

During wakefulness, the brain produces small choppy waves. As sleep progresses, the waves become slower and much larger. The waves during dream sleep resemble the chaotic, random activity of wakefulness. Brain waves are recorded in a document called an *EEG*, which stands for *electroencephalogram*, meaning the recording produced by measuring brain waves.

Figure 5.2   Brain activity

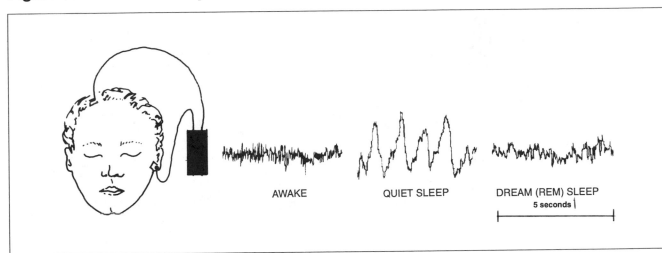

Figure 5.2.A The technician applies several electrodes to the scalp to measure and record brain activity.

Applying electrodes to the eyes to record eye movement

When a person is awake, the eyes move frequently to observe the environment. As a person becomes drowsy, the eyes begin to roll slowly back and forth. As the person develops quiet sleep, the eyes are peaceful and don't move. When the person dreams, even though the eyelids are closed, the eyes begin to move back and forth even more strongly than during wakefulness. However, the eyes respond to dream events rather than the outside world. (See Figure 5.3.) These recordings are called *electrooculogram* or *EOG*.

Applying electrodes to the chin to record muscle tone

The technician places electrodes on the chin to measure whether muscles are tense or relaxed and thus to detect dreaming sleep. During dreaming sleep, your brain prevents the activity of most muscles by inhibiting their tension-paralyzing your muscles. The muscles are normally tense in awake, relaxed in quiet sleep, and extremely relaxed during dreaming. The recording is called an *electromyogram (EMG)*. (See Figure 5.4.)

Muscle tone and eye movement—clues to dream sleep

The electrodes placed around your eyes and near your chin are especially important, allowing the doctor to determine whether you are in dream sleep, called *rapid eye movement (REM) sleep*. During this stage of sleep, most dreams occur, your eyes flit back and forth, and the muscles for body movement are relaxed. The electrodes placed near the eye can detect movements of the eye, those on the chin detect muscle tension. The eye movements in dream (REM) sleep are very rapid—more rapid than we can voluntarily move during wakefulness. These movements come in bursts of several movements together fol-

Figure 5.3 Eye movements

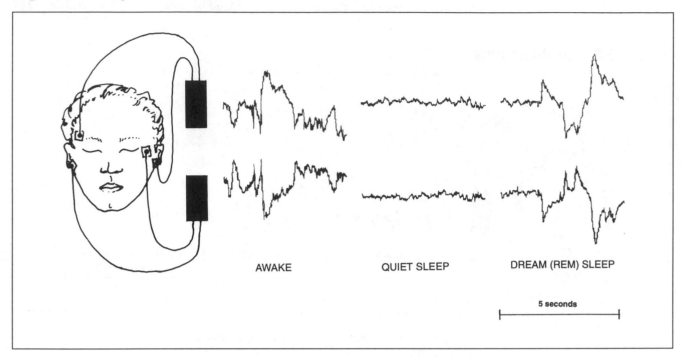

AWAKE   QUIET SLEEP   DREAM (REM) SLEEP

5 seconds

Figure 5.3   The technician places electrodes near the eyes to record signals representing eye movements. These signals control the movements of pens that write corresponding marks on the chart. This recording is called *EOG (electrooculogram,* record of electricity from the eye).

Figure 5.4 Muscle tension

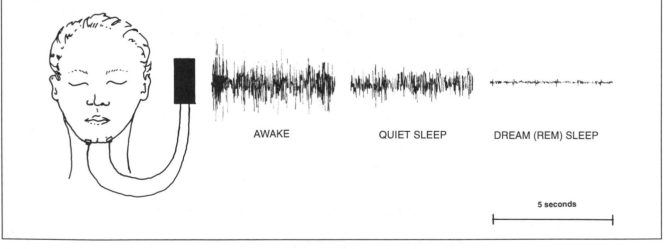

AWAKE   QUIET SLEEP   DREAM (REM) SLEEP

5 seconds

Figure 5.4   Two or three electrodes are placed on the chin to record muscle tension. The recording is called the *electromyogram (EMG).* The patterns of chin muscle tension shown are typical EMG signals which are characteristic of awake, quiet sleep, and dream sleep.

lowed by a period of seconds or minutes when the eyes are stationary. (See Figure 5.3 and Figure 5.4; see also Figure 6.4.)

Measurements of breathing effort and its effects

Air flow

The technician places devices at your nose and mouth to detect airflow and determine whether you are breathing. Each laboratory has a preferred measuring device, usually the thermistor, a small device sensitive to the alternate cooling and heating of air as it flows in and out of your mouth and nose. To see how these devices work, wet a finger and place it in front of your nose or mouth, then breathe in and out. You will feel a difference in temperature between the warm, moist air that you exhale and the cooler, dryer air that you inhale. If your breathing is interrupted, these devices will detect no temperature change. Air flow is sometimes also observed by measuring the increase in carbon dioxide in each exhaled breath. Air flow can help to identify normal breathing, partial obstructions, and the absence of breathing. (See Figure 5.5.)

If no air flows in or out for at least ten seconds, then we call the interruption an *apnea*. When breathing resumes after an apnea, there is an increase of breathing effort to make up for the lost breathing.

When airflow falls markedly but does not stop completely, then it is called *hypopnea*. Hypopneas are harder to measure than apneas and their significance is a matter of debate among doctors and sleep technicians.

Figure 5.5   Airflow

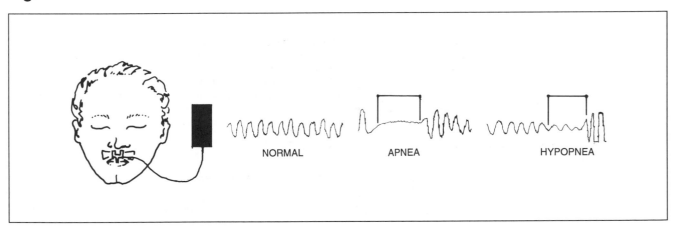

Figure 5.5   Temperature-sensitive thermistor tabs tell if air is flowing in and out of the nose. On the recording, *normal* breathing looks like a series of rounded hills. Going up the hill is breathing in, coming down is breathing out. About ten to fifteen breaths are recorded each minute, which is a normal rate. Also shown is an *apnea*—air does not flow and *hypopnea*—air flow is reduced.

Breathing effort

To establish whether the muscles that power breathing are active, the laboratory may use a wide, flat band that looks like a stretch bandage, belted around your chest as a measuring device. Another one may also be placed around your waist and abdomen as an additional measure of effort. To understand how these devices work, place one hand above your navel and the other on your chest, and breathe. Notice that your hands move each time you breathe in or out. The device produces a signal that indicates how much it is stretched by the expansion of the chest with each breath. In normal breathing, the effort of breathing creates a corresponding flow of air through the nose, but in obstructive apnea the flow is blocked despite the breathing effort. (See Figure 5.6.)

Figure 5.6　Breathing effort

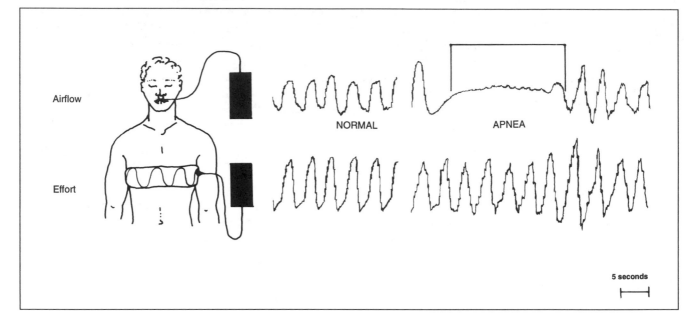

Figure 5.6　A belt around the chest measures the effort of the diaphragm and the expansion and contraction of the lungs, as seen in the lower tracing. The upper tracing shows the simultaneous airflow signal. During an obstructive apnea, there is no airflow present, but breathing efforts continue. During the apnea the effort appears to be less than during normal breathing, but this is because the airflow is blocked by the obstruction in the throat. When the airflow begins, there is an increased effort during recovery breathing.

Body position

Sometimes a position-sensitive device is used to indicate whether you are on your back or side, because some people show more or worse apneas when lying on their backs. (See Figure 6.8 which shows the record of positional apnea.)

Snoring

A specially modified microphone, similar to those used with tape recorders, is taped to the throat to measure snoring sounds. Snoring appears as bursts of activity on the polygraph tracing. Sound from the microphone and airflow from the thermistor are shown in Figure 5.7. In quiet breathing no sound is seen on the tracing. When snoring begins a burst of sound is recorded with each breath. During an apnea (a period without airflow), snoring ceases, since no air passes through the upper airway. When the obstruction ends, breathing and snoring both resume.

Figure 5.7   The sounds of sleep

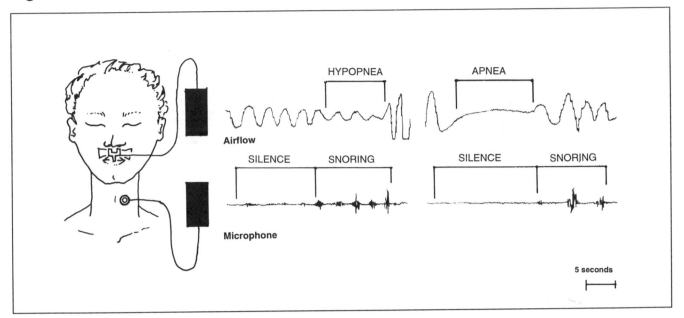

Figure 5.7   A microphone near the windpipe listens to the sounds of breathing. In the first panel breathing is quiet with normal airflow and no snoring for the first four breaths. Then snoring appears as a burst of sound with each breath. In the second panel, snoring has stopped, not because breathing is normal, but because an apnea has occurred.

Oxygen levels

A small device resembling a clothespin or a bandage will be placed on your fingertip (or attached to your earlobe) to measure the saturation or amount of oxygen in your blood. These devices, called *oximeters*, shine a red light through your finger or earlobe. Blood full of oxygen will be bright red; blood lacking in oxygen will be a darker red. The sensor detects changes in color, signaling how much oxygen is in your blood at any moment. Changes in oxygen level may be caused by sleep apnea. During an apnea, breathing stops and the supply of fresh oxygen to the lungs and blood is stopped, but the heart keeps pumping blood to all tissues and organs. The oxygen in blood becomes depleted rapidly. After a delay of a few seconds, this lack of oxygen appears in the oximeter tracing. When you finally resume breathing, the oxygen level rises to normal until the next apnea, when it dips again. These short dips are called *desaturations*—because the blood is not fully saturated with oxygen—and are characteristic of SAS. Thus the oximeter tracing is a critical part of the evaluation. The tracing typically shows that the changes in blood oxygen saturation lag behind the changes in breathing. (See Figure 5.8.)

Heart

Discs with adhesive backing are placed on your chest to collect signals that show the heartbeat or rhythm (these records are called the *ECG* or *electrocardiogram*; see Figure 5.9). Changes in breathing effort and interruptions in breathing during sleep affect the heart; thus the heart signal is important to establish the seriousness of the medical complications that result from sleep apnea. The

Figure 5.8   Measuring oxygen in the blood

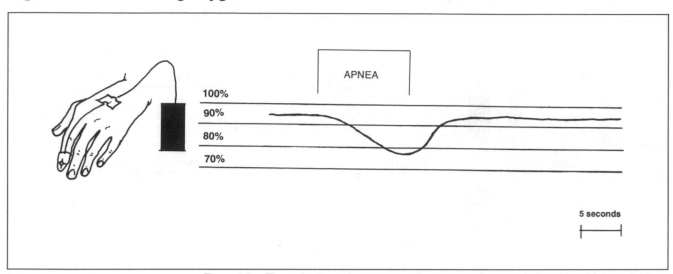

Figure 5.8   The *oximeter* probe measures the amount of oxygen in blood by shining a light through your finger.

extra effort of trying to breathe with a blocked airway usually causes changes in heart rate called *arrhythmias*.

Figure 5.9   The heartbeat

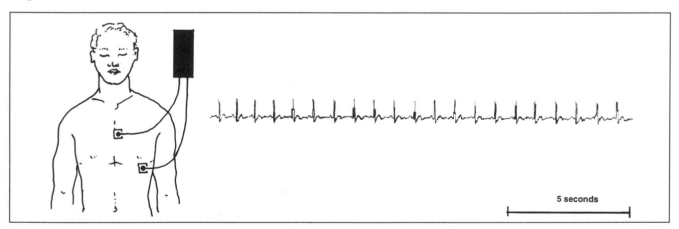

Figure 5.9   Electrodes record the heartbeat, producing the *electrocardiogram (ECG)*.

Leg movements

Electrodes may be placed on the legs to detect muscle twitching or jerking. Many apnea patiens exhibit such leg movements. In addition, another sleep condition (called *periodic leg movements* or *nocturnal myoclonus*) can be the cause of *excessive daytime sleepiness (EDS)*.

The study

Lights out

A trip to the bathroom before you retire is advisable, since getting in and out of bed will be a chore. The bedroom should be comfortable and as close to your home environment as possible. It will usually have an intercom system that you can use to summon the technician. You should feel comfortable about communicating freely with the technician so that your study can be accurate and useful. Generally, sound from the room is monitored continuously. Laboratories usually have a video camera that can record in low (or no) light conditions, perhaps with the aid of a red light. Depending on the laboratory, the bedding quality may range from utilitarian to the luxury of a five-star hotel.

In order to help the technician to check and calibrate the recording, you will be asked to open, close, and move your eyes and clench your teeth. When you go to sleep and during the night, the technician will ensure that the signals being recorded are of excellent quality so that the study can be interpreted correctly. The technician is trained to identify and correct the signals and to recognize false signals or *artifacts*. Like 'snow' on TV or static on the radio, artifacts are unrelated signals that the sensitive instruments pick up and trace.

The wires connected to you lead to a sophisticated amplifier and recorder in the hallway or separate control area. Most laboratories use paper recorders, which have several pens to create the *sleep study chart*. Each pen moves according to a signal from your body; all of the pens write on a wide, constantly moving band of paper. The technician watches the patterns the pens make on the paper and gets a good idea of how you are sleeping. Even the sound of the pens writing can tell an experienced technician when you are sleeping, dreaming, or waking. As you go to sleep, the busy, uncoordinated scratching of the pens slows and becomes regular and even. Some laboratories use computerized recording systems, which display lines on the computer monitor and record them on the computer instead of on paper.

Discovering the sleep apnea cycle

Although different patterns of breathing occur during the different stages of sleep, normal sleep shows no excessive disruption or interruption of breathing. The rate of breathing may change in different stages of sleep, but is rarely interrupted. Nothing obstructs or reduces the flow of air. The muscles that power breathing—the diaphragm and chest muscles—and those that keep the upper airway open work well to cause air to flow in and out of the lungs.

The sleep apnea cycle involves disruptions in sleep that show clearly in the brain activity summary of a person with SAS. Instead of the normal pattern of progression of brain waves that mark the several stages of sleep, the SAS sufferer has light sleep, periods of wakefulness, and little dreaming sleep. There are other related changes in the body. The sleep study chart can reveal if apnea is a source of sleep disruption.

Disordered breathing during sleep

In the laboratory, airflow is measured by sensors at the nose and mouth. To detect the recording of an apnea, the technician looks for evidence of air flowing in and out. If airflows stops for more than ten seconds, an apnea is present.

If the technicians discover an apnea, they will examine the tracing that shows the patient's effort to breathe. There are three categories of apneas: obstructive, central, and mixed. (See Figure 5.10 on page 53.)

Obstructive apnea

In *obstructive apnea,* the throat collapses so that when the sleeper tries to breathe, no air can flow. No breathing occurs because of a blockage or obstruction. Because there is evidence of a struggle to breathe, the apnea is classified as obstructive.

A typical obstructive apnea

The picture created in the laboratory shows that apnea dramatically affects sleep (Figure 5.10). The technician and the physician observe that an obstructive apnea involves changes in airflow, breathing effort, snoring sounds, oxygen levels, and heart rate. While it is true that the patient must repeatedly wake up because of apneas, at least enough to activate the muscles of the upper airway and remove the obstruction, usually it is not a total awakening or the awakening is too short to be remembered. Consequently, in the morning the sleep apnea sufferer feels fatigued and unrefreshed but cannot recall the hundreds of times that sleep was interrupted. This is the phantom nature of sleep apnea.

Central and mixed apnea

If, on the other hand, no efforts to breathe are observed and there is no airflow, the apnea is called central. A *central apnea* occurs when the sleeper's brain does not signal the muscles to create a breath. Although there is no blockage of the throat, there is no attempt to breathe.

Sometimes when breathing effort resumes after a central apnea, a blockage will occur. No airflow results because the throat is now blocked. These apneas are referred to as *mixed apneas* because they include elements of a central apnea and an obstruction. A mixed apnea is another form of obstructive apnea since it has a similar impact on the patient.

The technician will examine the other measurements for any record of the effects of the apnea on the patient. These additional measurements confirm that the interruption of breathing has significant consequences for the patient. Most apneas cause a decline in the concentration of oxygen in the blood, sometimes to extremely low levels. A significant apnea will show evidence in the brain waves of arousal of the brain and partial awakening by the patient. During the apnea the heart rate may fall and then rise abruptly as the obstruction is broken and the breathing resumes.

The multiple sleep latency test (MSLT)

Another test done in the sleep laboratory is called the *MSLT,* which measures how sleepy you are in the daytime by testing several times how long it takes you to fall asleep. Usually the MSLT is performed the day after an overnight study in the lab. It uses the same electrodes, and it's interpretation depends on the quantity and quality of the previous night's sleep.

Figure 5.10 Obstructive apnea

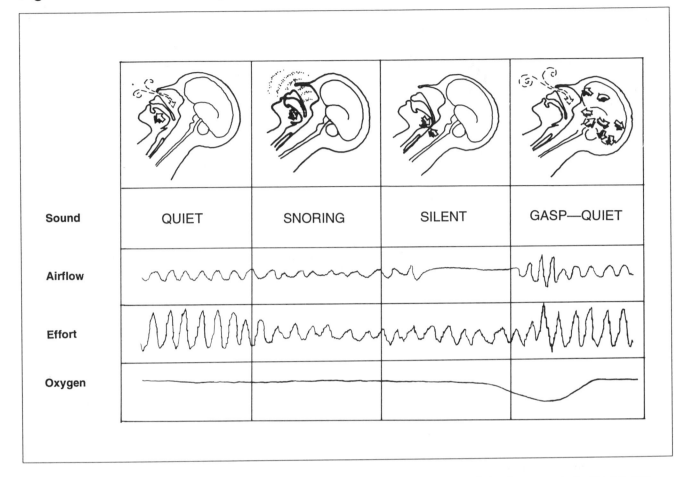

Figure 5.10 To the technician and the physician, an obstructive apnea looks like the combined tracings of airflow, effort, and oxygen saturation. A typical apnea shows changes in airflow, breathing effort, sounds, and oxygen levels. Silent breathing signals either normal sleep breathing or the awake condition. Diminished airflow caused by a partial obstruction or relaxation of the upper airway accompanies snoring. A complete blockage of airflow leads to silence, continued breathing effort, and a lowering of blood oxygen levels. Increased effort and the arousal of the brain open the throat, overcoming and breaking the blockage—heard as a gasp or snort. Higher levels of effort and airflow gradually subside as the oxygen levels rise.

The MSLT requires you to take four or more naps, separated by two-hour intervals, beginning at 9:00 or 10:00 A.M. The technician will have you go to bed and ask you to fall asleep in 20 minutes. If you snooze, you will be allowed 15 minutes before you are awakened. The test is easy, although boring. Bring something to read or work on in between naps. But don't fall asleep unless you are asked to, since naps affect the test results.

The results of the MSLT tell how sleepy you are according to laboratory standards. The MSLT is also used to diagnose another sleep disorder, *narcolepsy*. Narcolepsy is a neurological disorder that is far less common than SAS, but shares many symptoms. If in addition to sleepiness you have brief episodes of sudden muscle weakness (which doctors call *cataplexy*), especially if the episodes are triggered by strong emotions such as laughing or crying, you may

Figure 5.11 Obstructive, central, and mixed apnea

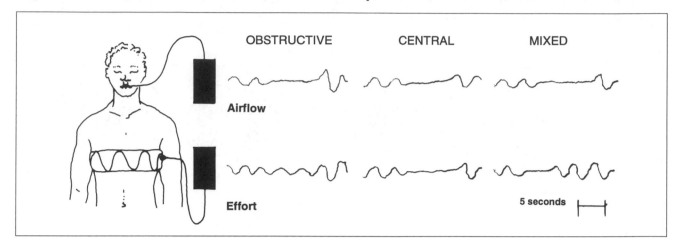

Figure 5.11   The obstructive apnea is caused by a blockage in the throat, although breathing effort continues. In the central apnea, however, the breathing effort ceases. A mixed apnea begins with a lack of breathing effort, but when breathing effort resumes, the throat may be blocked.

require an MSLT to help determine whether you have narcolepsy instead of or in addition to SAS.

If you have SAS to any degree, however, the results of the MSLT can be misleading. In a person with untreated SAS dreaming sleep appears within minutes of falling asleep, as would be seen in a patient with narcolepsy. Therefore, if you have SAS it may be necessary to treat the SAS for several weeks and then repeat the MSLT test before concluding that you have narcolepsy.

At-home sleep studies

Some laboratories have recently moved screening, diagnostic, and follow-up studies from the hospital into the patient's home because:

- A home study costs less than a hospital-based laboratory which has high overhead costs.
- New, reliable, safe, and portable electronic equipment can record data in the home.
- A home study can avoid the long wait for an appointment in some full-service sleep laboratories.
- A full-service sleep laboratory may not be available in your area.
- Some patients may have difficulty getting insurance coverage for a full-service sleep laboratory.

Advantages of home studies

Where available, home tests can be performed promptly, usually within a few days after the doctor orders them. Because any bedroom can serve as a sleep laboratory, scheduling depends only on the availability of equipment and the personnel to set it up properly, in your home or the office of the technician. The cost is usually less than that of a fully staffed sleep laboratory. But the greatest appeal for patients undergoing home study is the use of their own beds at their own homes. Sleep is highly personal and the 'fishbowl' effect of being in a hospital laboratory can unnerve some patients. If discomfort adversely influences their sleep, the test in the sleep laboratory becomes invalid because the study may not fairly represent the sleep problem. Except for the monitoring equipment, sleep in one's own bedroom is 'typical' and includes the favorable as well as unfavorable environmental influences that may be part of a sleep disorder. Home studies are well suited for follow-up testing to track the response of a patient to therapy as well as for screening and diagnosis.

Advantages of hospital laboratory studies

Both full laboratory sleep studies and a home studies have a role. The major benefits of hospital-based, technician-monitored sleep studies are flexibility and control. The laboratory usually can obtain more kinds of data in richer detail. Laboratory instruments are often more sensitive, elaborate, and comprehensive than portable recorders. A major responsibility of the technician monitoring the study is to ensure the quality of the data being recorded. If one of the measuring devices falls off, for example, the technician can immediately replace it. If an unusual signal appears in the tracing, the technician can track it down and eliminate it or identify its cause. This precision is helpful to the physician who will read the tests. On-the-spot troubleshooting means that a laboratory sleep study rarely has to be repeated because of technical errors. The technician makes observations during your night of sleep that can be invaluable in the interpretation of the polysomnogram.

The key to daytime fatigue

Thus we see the importance of viewing the sleep-wake cycle as one whole. The events (apneas) that disturb sleep are hidden from the sufferer. He or she is asleep and will rarely remember being aroused or awakened. Because sleep is culturally private, usually only a bed-partner or roommate might observe snoring and apneas, but they may not understand the significance of these events. The effects of disturbed sleep can be felt by the sufferer and observed by others during the day, however only recently have scientists been able to reveal the connection between disturbed sleep and waking behavior. Thus the sleep laboratory experience can close the loop and help explain daytime sleepiness and other symptoms. We observe sleeping to understand waking. In the following chapter the concepts and methods used by doctors and technicians to report on your sleep are covered in greater detail.

Chapter 6

Understanding your sleep report

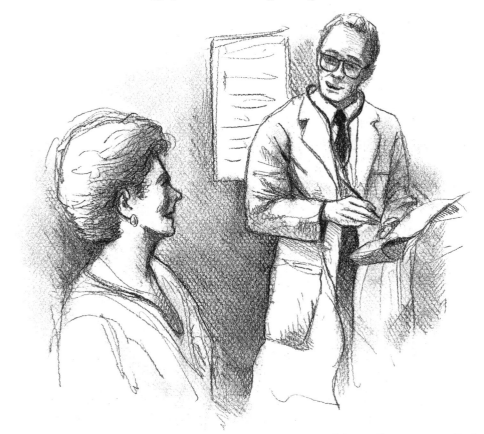

Your doctor can help you understand the meaning of your sleep study tests and decide how to overcome your problem.

Figure 6.1

Understanding makes a real difference

When I went for my first sleep study, I had some idea how signals from my body would be monitored, recorded, and interpreted to learn how well or badly I was sleeping. I knew that this information could help the doctors understand what was wrong and how to fix it. But I did not have a clear picture of the way that the test gathered information. Nor did I understand what the results meant. Thus I was anxious and confused as well as fatigued and irritable.

Perhaps if I had understood better what was supposed to happen, I could have gotten through the process with less worry. When I began to understand what is being done in the sleep laboratory and the meaning of my tests, I could stop feeling like a helpless subject and begin feeling empowered as a full participant in the recovery process.—J.H.

Your sleep study report

What the recordings mean

After capturing a detailed record of your brain waves, breathing sounds and motions, the technician and physician must analyze the vast amount of information. This complicated science of interpretation requires years of study and experience to master. The following basic introduction may help you to better understand the conclusions reached by your physician, but you can certainly read the rest of this book and carry out your treatment even if you don't read the rest of this chapter.

The final report prepared by the sleep laboratory will consist of the hypnogram as well as numerous calculations based on your sleep and breathing observed during the sleep study. The most important of these are:

- *Sleep efficiency*—the percentage of time in bed that you slept. In the normal person this number is at least 90%, i.e. 90 percent of the time in bed was spent in sleep.

- *Sleep latency*—the number of minutes it took you to fall asleep. It is a measure of how sleepy you are.

- *Percent of stages*—tabulates what percentage of the night you spent in each stage. These percentage distributions vary with age and also are affected by sleeping in the laboratory. In general, 50 to 60 percent of the night is in stages one and two, 10 to 15 percent is in stages three and four, while 20 to 25 percent is in dream sleep.

- *Apnea index (AI)*—the number of apneas observed per hour of sleep. Normal is defined as less than five apneas per hour, and over 10 in an hour is definitely abnormal.

- *Apnea plus hypopnea index (AHI)*—most laboratories also count hypopneas, particularly if they cause arousal from sleep and have an associated fall in oxygen saturation. This combined measure may be a better reflection of sleep disturbance and severity of sleep apnea than the apnea index.

- *Number of oxygen desaturations*—the number of times that the oxygen level decreased, usually by more than four percent. This is an indicator of apnea severity.

Your diagnosis and treatment plan

If you have SAS, some degree of partial or complete obstruction of your breathing occurs while you sleep, causing your sleep to be of poor quality. There are several ways of categorizing and evaluating SAS. The information in this chapter can help you to understand the process by which your sleep laboratory technician and doctors have identified your problem and help you to understand the way in which therapy can restore your sleep and health. Depending on how severely your sleep is disturbed, how badly the SAS affects your health overall, and how much the lack of sleep affects your daily well-being, there are several different treatment options that you and your doctors can choose. SAS is not something you should ignore—it won't go away by itself. However, there are effective treatments, and some combination of them should be able to provide you with at least partial, if not full, relief and restore your health.

The patterns of normal sleep

While doctors and scientists working at the forefront of knowledge about sleep may feel that we have just begun to open a few windows on how we sleep and wake, nevertheless the knowledge already won is truly impressive and interesting. This knowledge can be used to diagnose and treat persons suffering from some sleep disorders with results that sometimes seem miraculous.

The organization of behavior into awake and asleep, including dream sleep, has been observed for millennia. The course of sleep itself can now be understood in much greater detail. If we liken good sleep to a beautiful, harmonious symphony, we can appreciate the different movements and melodies of good sleep by studying the information from a sleep study. And, although only a qualified and trained physician or technician can determine if your sleep is in tune and thus good sleep, or out of tune, you can readily recognize and appreciate the difference. If your doctor is like an orchestra conductor or music critic, you can be an appreciative audience after this short course in sleep appreciation.

Clear patterns emerge when we look at short samples of recording over a time span less than a minute that allow us to classify the recording segment as one of the the six notes or stages of sleep and awake. Over a span of 90 minutes we see a tune or melody made up of pattern of these notes or stages of sleep and awake. And over the span of several hours during a night's sleep, we see a symphony consisting of repeats of the basic melody.

The melody of sleep

The stages of sleep are the notes. The stages of sleep follow a typical progression and pattern, much like the notes of a song. A single tune or sleep cycle lasts about 90 minutes. It begins with light, quiet sleep (stages one and two), goes on to deep quiet sleep (stages three and four), and then jumps to dream sleep. (See: Figure 6.2: The melody of sleep on page 60).

Figure 6.2   The melody of sleep

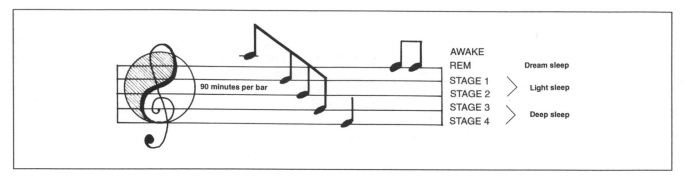

Figure 6.2   The melody of sleep follows a typical progression and pattern, much like the notes of a song.

The symphony of sleep

The sleep melody is repeated several (four or five) times during the course of a night's sleep. However, there are minor variations on the melody each time it is played. The balance between quiet sleep and dream sleep changes, so that each time the melody is repeated, there is more time spent in dream sleep. (See: Figure 6.3: The symphony of sleep on page 60)

Figure 6.3   The symphony of sleep

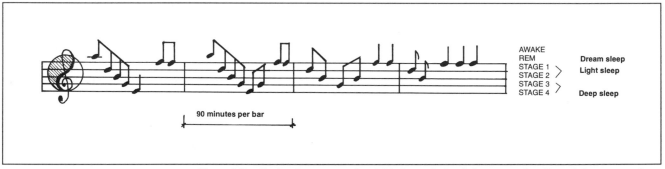

Figure 6.3   During the course of a night, the melody of sleep repeats with variations several times to form a symphony of sleep.

The normal pattern includes a wide range of differences among individuals. Many influences can interfere with this harmonious structure of sleep, including aging, drugs, alcohol, or depression. Sleep apnea fragments and disrupts the patterns of good sleep. A comparison with the patterns of a person with a sleep disorder can show dramatic differences, while in other cases the differences may be very subtle. Even though scientists aren't in agreement about how poor sleep causes each bad effect on daily life and health, we can say that if sleep looks normal, or can be made to look normal, the patient will feel good. Thus, if a person has abnormal sleep because of disordered breathing, and this breathing problem can be fixed, sleep may become normal and the patient can be restored to health.

Just as a trained musician and conductor can identify which instruments or group of instruments is playing out of order or out of tune and can teach the musicians how to make beautiful music together, so the sleep disorders specialist can identify the source of the disordered sleep and tell how to correct it.

Brain activity and the stages of sleep

For the several hours that you are being monitored, the continuous recording of brain waves provides information that can be analyzed to describe your sleep in more formal terms. Your doctor and the technician may discuss your sleep by referring to these categories. Normal sleep consists of periods of quiet, deep, sleep alternating with periods of dream sleep. Quiet, non-REM sleep usually occurs as one falls asleep and can be subdivided into four stages (stages one, two, three, and four). Usually there is a rapid descent from stage one through stage two into stage three and stage four. Each stage of sleep includes a mixture of EEG waveforms whose combination is used to identify that stage. Since these waveforms can be described in mathematical terms, computer programs can be used to analyze sleep records. But the brain waves alone are not sufficient and the specialist must also pay attention to eye movements, for example. We have seen how the sleep laboratory technician records several kinds of information about the sleeping person: brain activity, eye movements, muscle tension, snoring sounds, breathing effort, inspiration and expiration, oxygen in the blood, and heart rate. Let us look at a few seconds of each note or stage of sleep in Figure 6.4 to appreciate how the sleep specialist interprets this information.

Awake and drowsy

Brain waves are small, choppy, and disorganized when the patient is awake. Occasional eye movements and blinks occur and muscle tone is high.

With the eyes closed, a synchronized (alpha) rhythm begins and the EEG signal exhibits slower activity. The eyes may start to show a slow rolling back and forth motion.

Asleep

Stages one and two sleep

As the patient progresses from waking to stages one and two, brain waves show increasing strength and synchronization. Instead of the numerous small choppy waves characteristic of wakefulness, larger rhythmic waves build up. Giant EEG waveforms called *K complexes* and bursts of fast EEG activity called *spindles* are characteristic of stage two sleep. Slow movements of the eyes in a back and forth pattern, reminiscent of someone watching a tennis match, dominate state one but disapear as stage two develops.

Stages three and four (delta) sleep

Because of the prominence of delta waves in stages three and four, these stages are called delta sleep. Muscle tone in quiet sleep is diminished but present to a mild extent. Eye movements are absent—the 'wiggles' in the eye tracing during stage four in this example are actually the large delta waves from the brain showing up in the EOG.

Figure 6.4   The stages of sleep—recordings of the brain, eye, and muscles

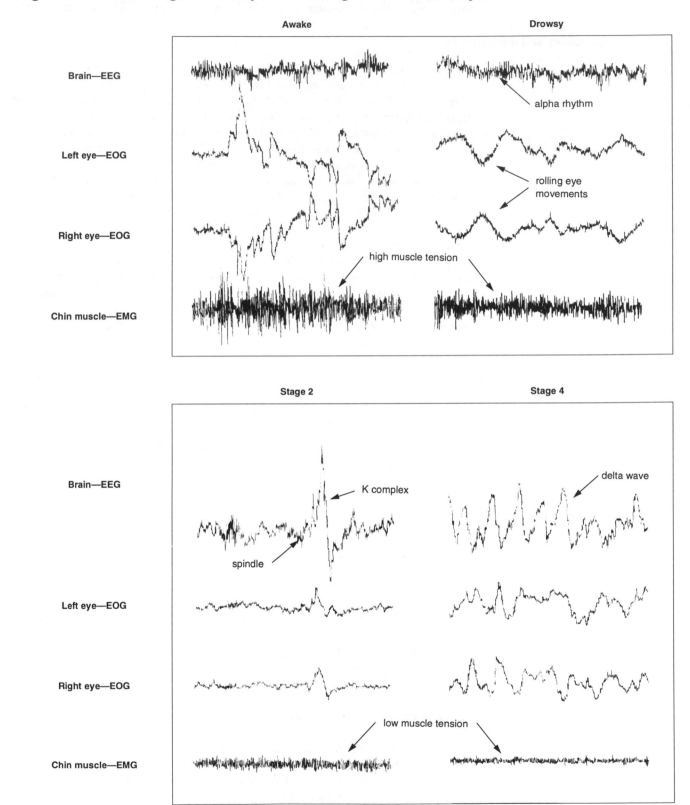

Figure 6.4   The stages of sleep—recordings of the brain, eye, and muscles

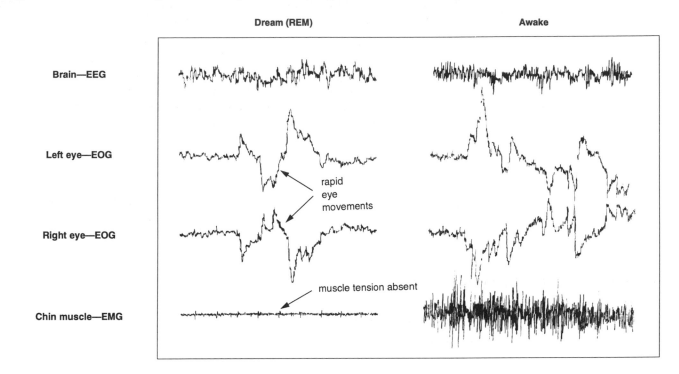

Figure 6.4   *Sleep stages* The awake and asleep condition and the stages of sleep can be recognized when the information from several channels of laboratory recordings is combined. The awake stage is repeated next to the dream stage for easier comparison.

Dream (REM) sleep

Dream (REM) sleep sharply contrasts with quiet sleep. The brain waves in REM sleep are random, almost as they appear in waking. In fact one cannot always be sure whether a patient is awake or in REM sleep based on the brain waves—so the information from the eye movements and the muscle tension is needed. A remarkable difference between dreaming and the other stages of sleep shows up in the electrodes that measure the eye motion. They record rapid flitting and repetitive eye motions, which often occur in bursts. The eye motions are more rapid than the eye movements of wakefulness. A person would find it difficult to mimic such rapid eye movements during wakefulness. At the same time that the eyes are active, the muscles of the trunk and limbs are very relaxed and indeed are effectively paralyzed.

The hypnogram

A diagram showing the stages of sleep for a night's sleep is called a *hypnogram* (sleep recording). It shows the symphony of the night and reveals the stages of sleep and their relationships in time. It is created by the technician who reviews and scores the recording made during a night of sleep. Each page of this overnight recording is 30 seconds long and is referred to as an *epoch*. Each epoch is examined for the characteristics of the EEG, EOG, and EMG and assigned a stage of sleep (wake, stages one through four, and REM). Since eight hours of sleep are 480 minutes and a page (epoch) of the record is half a minute, a total of 960 pages is produced for every eight hours of study. Once all the pages have been reviewed and assigned a specific stage of sleep, the results are graphed in the form of the hypnogram. (See Figure 6.5.) This is clearly an arduous, painstaking task requiring many hours of effort.

Recently, computers have been used to assist in finding patterns in the vast amounts of recorded information. Not only is the computer much faster and more efficient than a person, but it can analyze the information in even greater detail than can a person. However, the interpretation of the patterns must still be done by a skilled person. The examples were derived from studies generated by computer and confirmed by human scoring.

A normal sleep hypnogram

The stages of sleep from one night have been summarized in a normal hypnogram (See: Figure 6.5). Time from midnight to eight AM runs from left to right. Awake is at the top, and below it is displayed dream sleep (REM), and stages one through four. This normal person rapidly descended to stage four sleep,

Figure 6.5　A normal hypnogram

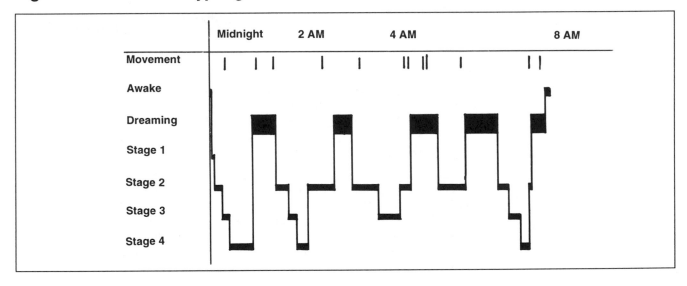

Figure 6.5　The orderly progression of the stages of sleep during the night typifies the normal hypnogram.

then had a brief period of dream sleep. Episodes of dream sleep became more frequent as the night progressed, but the last episode was quite brief. There was also a late period of stage four sleep about 7 AM which is not typical of normal sleep.

Disturbed sleep

How the sleep apnea cycle disrupts sleep

The trained technician or physician can identify the notes, the melody, and the symphony that make up normal, restorative sleep by recording and analyzing brain waves. Sleep disturbed by apnea can be readily identified because it does not show the same orderly progression typical of normal sleep. A person experiencing breathing problems during sleep will wake up or experience a micro-arousal. This awakening takes place because the center of the brain that controls sleep—the brain stem—generates activity in other parts of the brain while it is sending signals to reopen the airway. This connection between breathing and sleep is at the core of the problem for SAS patients.

The hidden connection between breathing and sleep

However, the connection between disordered breathing and poor sleep is hard for the non-specialist to recognize and was only recently understood by scientists. One factor that may hide this connection is the difficulty most people without special training may have in making a connection between events which take place on a short time scale, of about one or two minutes, and events which take time on a scale of several hours. The sleep apnea cycle takes about two minutes as the sufferer goes from quiet breathing, to snoring, to apnea, and then gasps and has a micro-arousal. Yet, these brief but frequent micro-arousals disrupt the pattern of sleep stages which take place in a normal cycle of about 90 minutes, repeated over eight hours. The great strides made in the last generation by scientists and physicians have bridged this difference in scale—two minutes compared to 90 minutes and eight hours—and clarified the connection between breathing and sleeping (See page 37). We know that the brain responds to breathing difficulties and thus snoring and thus SAS disturbs normal sleep. Today the laboratory technician and physician interpret the records of sleep in order to diagnose and treat SAS. Treatment is based on restoring the free flow of each breath. (See: Figure 6.6: The hidden connection between breathing and sleep on page 66).

During a typical two-minute sleep apnea cycle, changes take place in sound, airflow, breathing effort, and brain waves. If we examine the hypnogram and the brain wave frequency plot which summarize the events of the whole night, each two-minute cycle is barely legible at this scale. However, the chaotic picture of sleep stages is very different from the orderly progression seen in normal sleep.

The hypnogram (Figure 6.7: A hypnogram of sleep disturbed by apnea on page 67) illustrates a night of sleep for a patient with severe sleep apnea. Because of the breathing disorder and the frequent micro-arousals caused by it, sleep is very poor in quality. Compared to the normal hypnogram (Figure 6.5: A normal hypnogram on page 64), we see that the apnea patient experiences no deep sleep (stages three and four). Much more time is spent in waking and very little time is spent dreaming. And, hundreds of changes from one state to another occur. Neither the 90 minute melody nor the eight hour symphony are recognizable in this jumble of notes. No wonder the tired sleep apnea patient sleeps in the day at any opportunity.

Figure 6.6 The hidden connection between breathing and sleep

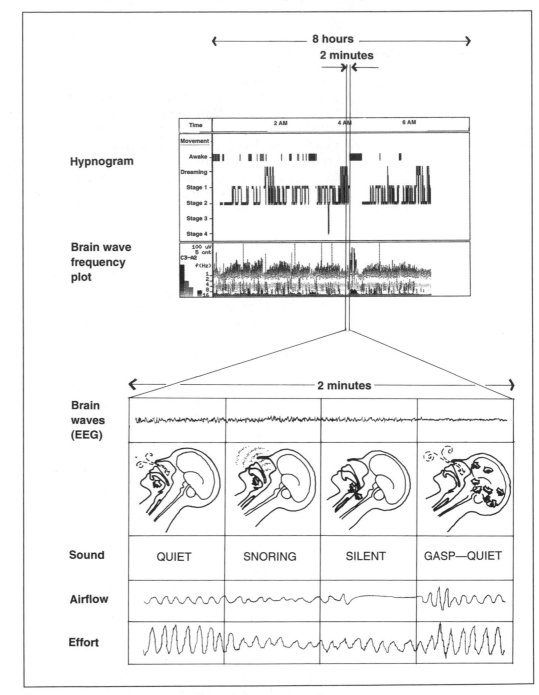

Figure 6.6   The sleep apnea cycle takes about two minutes. But it interrupts the normal pattern of sleep stages which repeats over a period of 90 minutes throughout the eight hours of sleep. Thus the short scale event of SAS—two minutes—is hidden in our perception of the night which is a much longer time period (240 two-minute SAS cycles in eight hours).

Effect of position

Some people have more severe apnea, or develop apnea, when sleeping on the back. A sensor may be attached to a belt around the chest which reports if the

Figure 6.7   A hypnogram of sleep disturbed by apnea

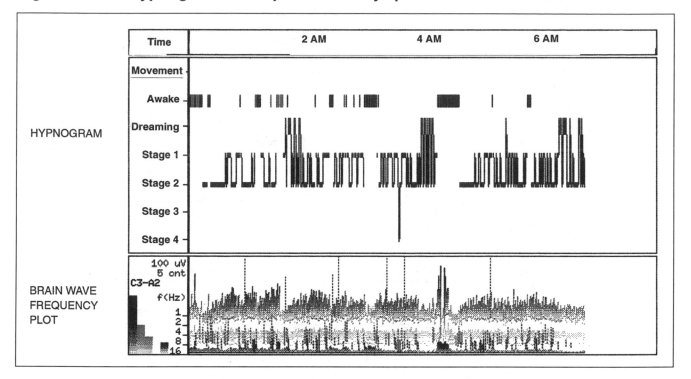

Figure 6.7   Frequent micro-arousals caused by SAS interrupt the orderly progression of sleep stages, practically eliminating deeper stages of sleep and dream sleep; the fuzzy pattern of the brain-wave plot confirms the absence of a normal cycle of quiet and dream sleep.

patient is lying on the back or side. A patient with this positional sensitivity may show more apneas and greater oxygen desaturation as measured by the oximeter when lying on his or her back. In the hypnogram shown in Figure 6.8, when the patient is on either the left or right side as shown in the middle panel, then there are fewer apneas and the oxygen saturation is higher. However, when he is on his back, then there are severe dips in the blood oxygen caused by more severe and more frequent apneas.

Before and after treatment for SAS

If disturbed breathing is the cause of poor sleep, then fixing the breathing should—and does—repair the sleep.

The remarkable return of normal sleep when a patient with sleep apnea syndrome is treated is demonstrated in before-and-after hypnograms (Figure 6.9). Before treatment, the sleeper had frequent awakenings and transitions between stages, many arousals, no delta sleep, and very little dreaming (REM) sleep. Thus, in the hypnogram the trained observer notes the poor cycling of quiet and dream sleep, the lack of deep sleep, and the presence of frequent awakenings. The brain-wave plot confirms this by showing a monotonous tracing. A fuzzy and damped-out pattern indicates an absence of the normal cycle of quiet and dream sleep during the night. There is no good music in this night—no pattern of a melody, let alone a symphony.

Figure 6.8   Positional apnea

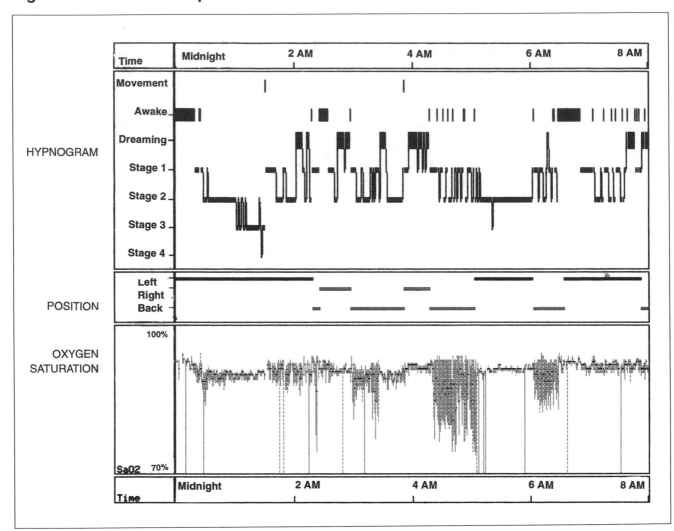

Figure 6.8   Apneas may be worse when lying on one's back, causing poorer quality sleep and reducing oxygen levels in the blood. The top panel (A) is the hypnogram, the middle panel (B) shows the plot of position: when the patient is lying on the left side, right side, or back. The bottom panel (C) shows oxygen saturation levels which fall when the patient is on his back.

During treatment with CPAP, however, this same patient has a dramatically different—and nearly normal—hypnogram. On this first treatment night, which included time to establish the correct pressure, the same patient with severe obstructive apnea (SAS) experienced excellent, restful sleep. The complete orchestral rendition of a night is clearly seen. As soon as adequate CPAP pressures were reached, there was a *rebound effect* or more than usual amount of quiet, slow-wave sleep and dreaming sleep. Dream sleep alternates with quiet sleep three times, with sharp contrasts between the two kinds of sleep on both the brain-wave plot and the hypnogram. Strong bands of deep, delta sleep alternate with abnormally prolonged dream (REM) sleep periods. The patient is exhibiting the intensity of sleep when sleep occurs after prolonged sleep deprivation. Because nasal CPAP therapy eliminates the sleep apnea which had interfered with sleep, this patient is able to breathe and sleep normally for the first time in years.

Figure 6.9   Before and after treatment for apnea

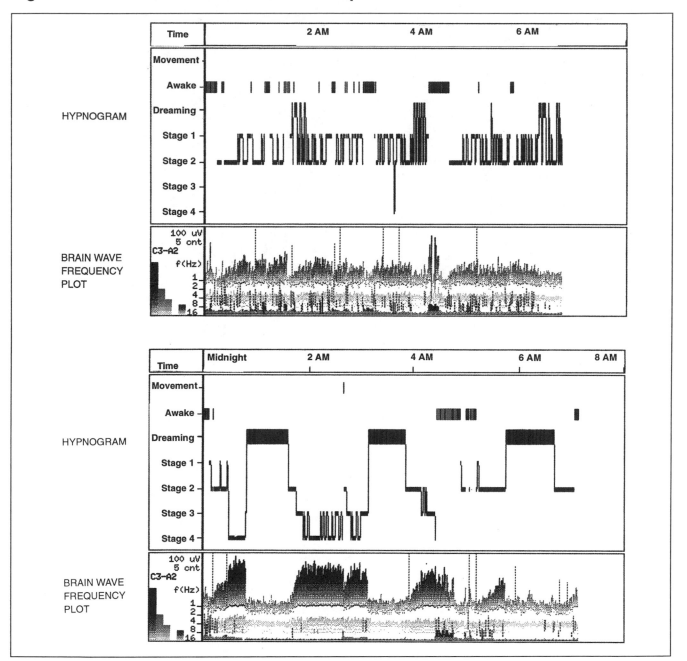

Figure 6.9.A The person with untreated apnea has disturbed sleep. In the hypnogram, the trained observer notes the poor cycling of quiet and dream sleep, the lack of deep sleep, and the presence of frequent awakenings. A fuzzy and damped-out pattern indicates an absence of the normal cycle of quiet and dream sleep during the night. There is no good music in this night—no pattern of a symphony, let alone a melody.

Figure 6.9.B During the first night of CPAP treatment for apnea a near-normal pattern of sleep is shown in both the hypnogram and the display of brain wave frequency. The complete orchestral rendition of a good night's sleep is clearly seen. As soon as adequate CPAP pressures were reached, there was a *rebound* (more than the usual amount) of quiet, slow-wave sleep and dreaming sleep. The patient is exhibiting the intensity of sleep when sleep occurs after prolonged sleep deprivation.

Chapter 7

The miracle of relief

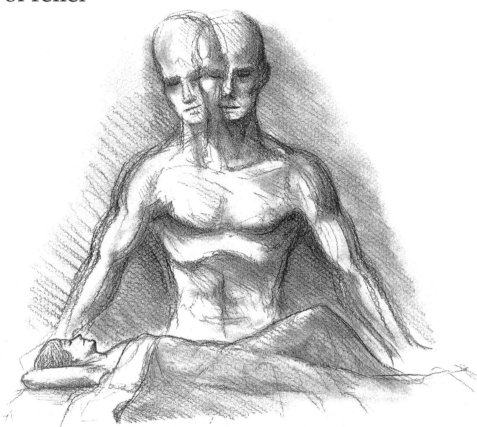

An immediate change came over her countenance. *Her breathing suddenly became quiet and regular. Gone was the inefficient rocking and heaving of chest and abdomen. In its place was a quiet regular motion of the chest in concert with the abdomen. She was breathing without interruptions by apneas. And her brain waves had lost the busy, chaotic look of the awake brain and were settling into the even, smooth patterns of the sleeping brain; they were rolling like offshore waters—regular steady swells that lift a boat gently and set it down again. She was truly asleep for the first time in ten years.—TSJ*

Figure 7.1

Me and my CPAP

I have a very intimate relationship with my CPAP machine. I don't really like it, but I wouldn't go anywhere without it, and I take it to bed with me nightly. Getting along with it isn't easy—I have to change its filter, wash its hoses, clean and adjust the mask. It's as much work as a pet. But if I am getting along well with the machine, I will sleep well and feel good the next day, so I must keep it happy.

Sometimes the noise of the blower and the air rushing into the mask annoys me. But this 'white noise' insulates me from traffic and other noises that might wake me. It took me a long time to get used to my CPAP machine, but when I put it on I am asleep practically within seconds, as if it were a soporific, and if I try to sleep without it I don't feel right.

I don't look glamorous wearing the mask, but I also wasn't very appealing when I snored. I used to feel embarrassed about using the mask but I realized that the CPAP is only a prosthesis that helps me overcome a small defect in my body so that I can sleep well. Many people wear glasses without embarrassment despite equally trivial defects in their eyes. Sometimes I imagine I am an astronaut, suiting up for my nightly dream-walk.

When I travel with the CPAP machine, people sometimes ask what it is, which is an opportunity to talk about sleep. Having this device makes me an expert on sleep, and nearly everyone has some problem sleeping. In fact, as one friend remarked, I have an advantage over most people—I finally do know how to sleep.

A great catalogue of new mask styles includes custom-made masks. In fact, new models of CPAP are coming out that are said to be smaller, lighter, quieter, more suitable for traveling—I can't wait to try them. I think I'll keep using my CPAP machine.—J.H.

What is CPAP?

Individuals with SAS cannot breathe while asleep—the soft, pliable tissues of the throat collapse during sleep, and block the flow of air into the lungs. Suppose there were a way to keep the throat from collapsing—so that the air could flow. Wouldn't that solve the breathing problem and allow one to breathe and sleep at the same time? But what can we put into the throat during sleep? The answer is air blown in with a bit of additional pressure. Air with a positive pressure (force) applied to the upper airway during sleep can prevent the recurring collapse of the throat, thereby eliminating the obstruction of breathing and the resulting disruption of sleep. Positive pressure therapy has restored normal sleep to a growing number of patients.

Dr. Colin Sullivan, an Australian pulmonologist, first used CPAP in 1981 to treat obstructive sleep apnea. *CPAP* stands for *continuous positive airway pressure:* the pressure within the upper airway is maintained positive (higher than the surrounding atmospheric pressure) by this device, continuously. CPAP (pronounced "see-pap") requires a portable, quiet electrical device from which a six-foot (two-meter) hose leads to a mask, which is held to the patient's nose by an adjustable harness. As you put on the mask, the flow of air is like a spring zephyr of about 15 to 20 miles per hour, about right for sailing or like what you might feel riding a bicycle. At first, it seems that no one could sleep with such a device blowing air into one's face, and it does take getting used to. However, the flow of air quickly drops to provide approximately enough to match each breath, and most people soon adjust to the feeling—if any—of pressure.

Hundreds of thousands of patients (an estimated 300,000 through 1992) have experienced their first good sleep in years when this therapy was applied in the sleep laboratory. The majority of them use it nightly for years and enjoy normal sleep. CPAP therapy is more likely to succeed if the patient fully understands how it works, monitors the treatment to make many small adjustments, and does the maintenance that assures effective treatment. In this book, as in discussions with your doctor and others familiar with sleep disorders, you will find *CPAP* used in more than one sense: as the name of a type of machine as well as referring to the treatment using one or another of these machines.

How does CPAP work?

The air under positive pressure acts as a *pneumatic splint* to keep the airway open during inhalation and exhalation, preventing the airway from collapsing. Thus the CPAP device breaks the cycle of sleep–obstruction–apnea–awakening and allows the wearer to sleep without interruption. Although the patient may worry about gasping for air or having a strong wind blowing into the nose, a properly fitted mask is not uncomfortable and the air pressure is easy to get used to. Rarely has the amount of pressure caused any problems when properly and carefully applied. The pressure is much lower than when we sneeze, and rarely enough to cause ears to 'pop' as they might in flight. Sometimes the patient is so exhausted and irritable from months or years without proper sleep that even a properly fitted mask seems overwhelming. But this emotion quickly fades when the patient experiences good sleep.

What is a nasal CPAP unit?

Small differences exist among machines from different manufacturers. (A typical CPAP in use is shown in the illustration page 81; also see Appendix D on page 139.) The CPAP device in its simplest form consists of:

- a soft, pliable mask that fits over the nose; or a device that holds a flexible, cushioned tube against or in each nostril
- straps or other headgear to keep the mask in place
- a fan or turbine to pressurize air
- a control system to maintain the pressure at a designated level
- a hose to connect the blower unit to the nasal mask.

These components have been refined since 1983, when the devices became available commercially. The fans, once noisy belt-driven blowers, are now quiet, rapidly responding turbines functioning with direct drive and electronic control of motor speed. The masks come in several sizes and shapes, made of softer, more comfortable, and longer lasting material. The headgear is more comfortable and easier to adjust and to apply to fit a variety of head shapes and sizes. Finally, the external pressure valve has now been superseded by automatic circuits to monitor and control the pressure. The modern CPAP device is smaller, lighter, quieter, and easier to use. CPAP units are now highly portable and adaptable to 220-, 110-, 24-, and 12-volt power sources. Travel with CPAP has never been easier and many patients who use CPAP will not leave home without it.

Trial and titration of CPAP in the laboratory

Applying pressure and observing results

In the sleep laboratory you will be fitted with a CPAP mask and the measuring electrodes. A small amount of air flow is established to allow comfortable breathing. Once you have gone to sleep and exhibit recurrent apneas with obstruction, the technician increases the pressure in the mask.

The air pressure applied through the mask to your nose is measured by a thin tube from a hole in the mask to a meter, either a water manometer or an electronic pressure sensitive device. A water manometer is a U-shaped tube partly filled with water that measures the difference in pressure between air pressure and another pressure such as the CPAP pressure delivered to your mask. This difference is determined by observing how high the measured pressure raises a column of water in the manometer tube. Typical air pressure for treating apnea might be 10 centimeters of pressure, which you would create by drinking through a straw that reached 10 cm. (3.9 inches) from the top of the drink to your mouth. Conversational speech is created by air pressure of about seven cm. past the vocal cords, as reported by Robert T. Sataloff (*Scientific American*, December 1992).

The technician or doctor increases the pressure gradually until the obstructive apnea cycle is broken. Laboratories may vary in their standard procedures, but the principle is the same. When the apneas have been eliminated, your breathing and heart rate become regular and you rapidly descend into deeper stages of sleep. Further adjustments in the pressure may be needed as the night progresses. As you enter REM sleep or change to an unfavorable position (such as on your back) more pressure may be needed to prevent apneas. The response of the upper airway to changes in pressure is poor until some minimum threshold pressure is reached; then, the response is more sensitive (Figure 7.2 on page 75). As the pressure approaches the effective level, increases in pressure open the obstruction and progressively eliminate partial obstructions and snoring. The patient immediately begins to sleep without disturbance. Your correct pressure must be carefully established during testing and maintained with equal care and accuracy in home treatment. The technician notes the appropriate pressure and you sleep the remainder of the night with CPAP in place. You may have many vivid dreams from the *rebound effect*. When a person who has not slept well for some time can sleep deeply, a greater than usual amount of dream sleep occurs, as if the mind needs to catch up on dreaming. (For a more technical presentation of sleep before and after treatment by CPAP, see Before and after treatment for SAS on page 67 in Chapter 6.)

Figure 7.2   How CPAP works

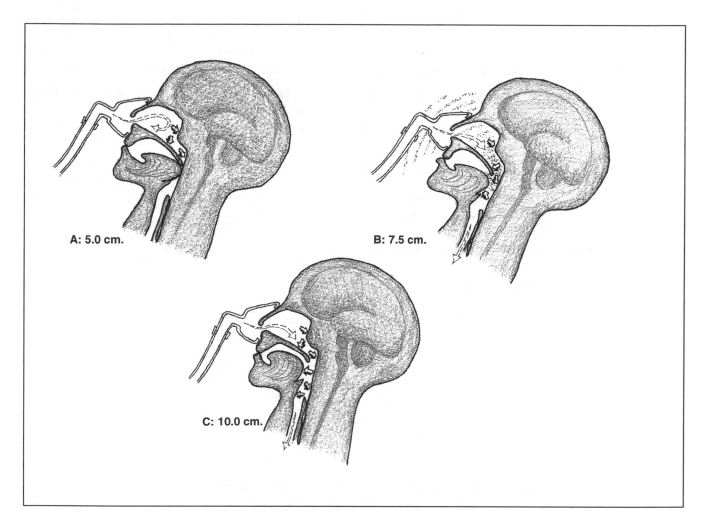

A: 5.0 cm.

B: 7.5 cm.

C: 10.0 cm.

Figure 7.2   Air blowing into the nose under pressure holds open the upper airway and prevents snoring and apnea. The application of positive air pressure keeps the airway from collapsing. The pressure increases (from 5 cm., to 7.5 cm., and finally to 10 cm.). The airway is progressively opened by the additional pressure until the apneas, hypopneas, and snoring are eliminated. At 5 cm. (A) there is not enough pressure to overcome the obstruction. At 7.5 cm. (B), the obstruction has been opened but persistent snoring shows that more pressure is needed. With the addition of more pressure (A), 10 cm. total pressure permits free breathing. Precise titration takes all night because the technician has to establish the lowest pressure that will eliminate the problems in various sleep positions, quiet sleep, dreaming sleep, and late as well as early in the night.

In the morning following a trial of CPAP, you may feel remarkably well rested and eager to use CPAP again as soon as possible. For many patients, a prescription for CPAP at the prescribed level can be written the day after the overnight study. In other cases, the information from your test may require additional study before a decision can be made. Unfortunately, some labs have such a backlog of unread tests that you may have to wait.

Obtaining a CPAP for your home use

The delivery of CPAP devices for home use usually starts when the physician notifies a local home care company (which specializes in the provision and maintenance of medical equipment to the home) that CPAP is required, and prescribes the amount of pressure. The laboratory may provide information about mask size and other information useful for fitting the mask to the patient. Most home care companies will go into the home with the equipment and supplies necessary to fit the patient correctly. Then the home care company delivers the unit to your home, fits the mask, sets the pressure correctly, tests the unit and reviews details of use with the patient and his or her family.

Discuss your needs and the available options with the therapist from the home care company. The therapist should troubleshoot during the time you are using CPAP; however, the willingness and competency of these companies to offer help and expertise varies considerably.

If you have problems and questions, call your therapist. Your doctor depends on the home care company to fill your prescription as a pharmacy would dispense medications. You may also contact the laboratory technician or your doctor for help.

Other devices and features for treatment

The bi-level pressure treatment device

Patients whose treatment requires high pressure may benefit from an effective new method that can reduce overall pressures. This more complex machine for the delivery of positive pressure is called a bi-level device or *BiPAP®*, which stands for *bi-level positive airway pressure*. Bi-level devices can provide two different pressure levels, for inhalation and exhalation. For example, instead of a constant pressure of 10 cm. with CPAP, with bi-level positive airway pressure, a patient might receive 10 cm. on inhalation but only five cm. on exhalation. Apnea may thus be controlled with lower pressures, and patients who found CPAP difficult to tolerate might be able to use a bi-level device.

Despite the greater expense of bi-level devices compared to CPAP, nevertheless for some patients the more complex functions and features of the bi-level devices provide worthwhile benefits, and are now reimbursed in over half the states by Medicare and Medicaid.

Some bi-level devices including the *BiPAP®* can also provide a timed function to treat central or mixed apneas. If the patient's breathing stops for longer than a predetermined interval, the device will deliver the inspiration level of pressure, in effect initiating and partially supporting breathing for the patient.

Ramp function

A recent development in CPAP has been the addition of a *ramp* function, which is also called *adjustable pressure delay* (APD), into the control system for the unit. The ramp allows the prescribed CPAP pressure to be achieved slowly, rising along a ramp instead of starting at the ultimate pressure. Some machines offer a range of ramp times, from no delay to forty-five minutes; the ramp time may be preset or may be adjusted by the patient or a technician. A gradual buildup of pressure may be more comfortable. In fact the patient may be asleep before full pressure is achieved. The ramp approach is similar to the sleep lab, where the technician increases pressures after the patient has fallen asleep. Patients highly tolerant of CPAP do not find the ramp necessary, however.

The next generation of CPAP machines

Soon we will see a new generation of CPAP machines. These 'smart' machines will respond to the needs of the patient for pressure rather than always delivering air at a fixed pressure. For example, when the patient is lying on the back, or in dream sleep, a higher pressure would be delivered. When breathing is free of obstruction, the pressure would fall. Patient comfort and acceptance will be vastly better and it is possible that CPAP titration will no longer be required.

An important relationship deserves patience

Not everyone responds immediately and dramatically to CPAP treatment; response may be gradual. But be patient. More than 300,000 people in the United States switch on their CPAP unit every night, inviting this machine to sleep with them despite its inconveniences. And, although the relationship between patient and machine has elements of hate, love triumphs when dawn arrives after a good night's sleep. As in any other viable relationship, both partners must work hard to adjust to and accept the frailties of the other. The manufacturer, home care company, sleep specialists, laboratory technicians, other patients, and support groups can help to make your CPAP machine suitable for your use. You are responsible for making adjustments in your life to derive the most benefits from CPAP therapy.

Some patients may hesitate to accept treatment for SAS because they wonder if the treatment might create problems. CPAP treatment for SAS has been undertaken only since 1981 so there is not a large population that has been using it for a long time. No research on the benefits or risks of the long-term use of CPAP has been published. We have some information that untreated SAS increases mortality (people with untreated SAS die sooner) and it is believed that treating SAS with CPAP reduces the risk of premature death. If it were established that the use of nasal CPAP prevented heart attacks, strokes, and premature death, then the daily inconvenience of the machine's use would perhaps be more tolerable. In fact, medical scientists do have preliminary evidence that CPAP can prolong life, especially in those severely affected patients with greather than 20 apneas per hour of sleep. Tracheostomy has also been associated with improved survival in the most severely ill patients, but other surgical procedures have not yet been proven to favorably influence longevity. Population studies currently taking place in the U.S., Israel, and Scandinavian countries should answer questions about the benefits of nasal CPAP.

Meeting your preferences and needs

The competitive marketplace has driven several manufacturers to develop many CPAP machines. These companies have responded rapidly to the needs of physicians and patients. The results are better, quieter, more comfortable, and more reliable units. The cost of devices, however, has steadily risen with the general rise in health-care costs.

Most home care companies offer equipment made by one manufacturer, which allows the company to acquire experience with a limited number of models. This relationship, however, limits the possibilities for the patient, at least when the prescription is first filled. Despite the diversity of available models, the patient (the consumer) rarely has the opportunity to pick and choose. If you were to attend a professional meeting of sleep researchers and practitioners you could see exhibits by manufacturers of CPAP units. The manufacturers' representatives will demonstrate the latest CPAP machines, headgear, and face masks to anyone. The attendees, however, are usually not sleep apnea sufferers. Patients need a fair in which they could examine the range of CPAP equipment to get an idea about most suitable designs. As a partial response to this need for information, we have illustrated equipment and accessories used in evaluation and treatment in Appendix D on page 139. The illustrations and information were provided by courtesy of the manufacturers and have been selected to show the range of resources available to the patient, and is not a complete showing of the currently available equipment.

Patients using CPAP for some time with persistent problems that care providers have not solved are interested in learning about better solutions. If you are persistent, you can solve nearly any type of problem of comfort and function. Until patients have experienced treatment, they cannot know what type of headgear or mask, for example, would be most comfortable. Most accessories such as masks can be used with CPAP devices from any manufacturer. In some parts of the United States, home care companies operate retail outlets where patients can examine several models of CPAP machines and masks. You may be able to rent a device for a month to determine if it is suitable, and later purchase it. You could call several home care companies to learn about the models they handle, their support and services, and their billing procedures. You can try different models to determine levels of noise, comfort, and other important features. As a consumer of health-care services, you must be prepared to communicate to your doctor and home care service that you require comfort and satisfaction. You and your doctor may choose another unit or company if one is not satisfactory. Certain arrangements, such as a list of accepted vendors that your HMO or insurance company has established, may limit your choices.

Education, information, and consumer choice in matters open to individual preference make it easier for the patient to take full advantage of CPAP therapy. Clearly, the health-care system, manufacturers, home care companies, insurers, and patients all have an interest in further improvements. Patient support groups such as AWAKE exchange information about devices and techniques, including equipment from various manufacturers. Patients are eager to share their own tricks of the trade to help each other get the best from equipment and services.

Who should not use CPAP?

Although extremely safe, nasal CPAP should not be used by some patients. The force of the air that is holding the throat open also pushes against other structures. Theoretically, a weakened part of the lung, as emphysema patients might have, could rupture under the air pressure. A chronic sinus or ear condition could worsen since pressure in the upper airway might impede drainage. These contraindications, or reasons not to use the therapy, are uncommon and rarely prevent the use of nasal CPAP. Yet, it is important to be aware of them and to discuss your questions with your doctor.

Sleep is the basis for life

At its best, CPAP provides quiet, restful sleep uninterrupted by apneas. Most importantly, symptoms such as excessive daytime sleepiness, frequent awakenings at night, or loud snoring should be cured. Your bed partner should also sleep better, because the noise of the CPAP is quieter than your snoring. Your bed partner's anxiety from listening for your breathing to start after each apnea should disappear.

During the first few days and weeks of use, if the device is working effectively your body will restore the sleep that you have lost for many years. Your sleep will be deeper, with increased amounts of REM and delta sleep. As a result, you will awaken feeling truly refreshed. Your days will be more productive and you will have a new-found source of energy. Decisions that were difficult to make or that you put off will be easier to face. Friends and colleagues will notice a big change, particularly in your mood. Your spouse and relatives will comment that you are more like your old self.

You may want to keep a daily log or diary of your sleep and activities, including changes in your outlook, general well-being, and relationships. Not only will this log help you to pinpoint possible problems in therapy, but you will be recording your recovery. You may discover specific problems that disappear when you recover and thus help to identify additional problems that untreated SAS may cause.

If you have not joined a support group or talked with other SAS patients, now is the time. You are part of a small group of travelers who have been in a land of constant fatigue and are now returning to the land of normal sleep, experiencing the wonder and joy of life. Chapter 8 reviews how to overcome problems with CPAP and how you can improve your use of this lifesaving therapy.

Chapter 8

Making CPAP work for you

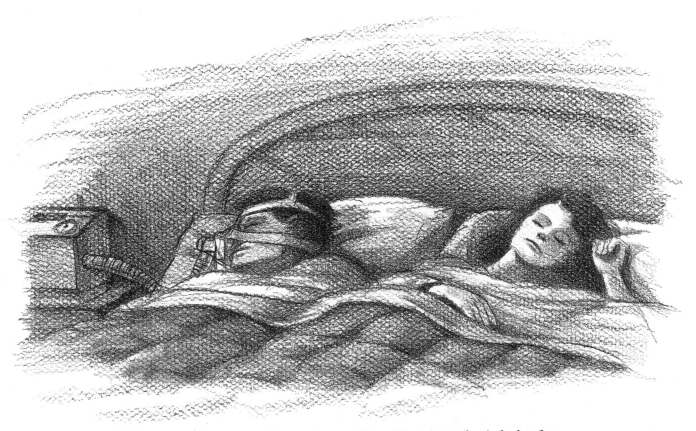

There is nothing like a good night's sleep.

Figure 8.1

How I learned to make CPAP work for me

CPAP therapy should work without problem, and for the majority of patients, it is simple and provides relief. Most treatment moves along without difficulty and with relief for the patient. Patients can overcome nearly any obstacle to success. There is nothing like a good night's sleep, and for people with SAS, making CPAP work is well worth any inconvenience or effort.

However, I have a different story to tell. I am sure that Murphy's Law, "If anything can go wrong, it will," is true. After many months I have solved the problems, with the aid of technicians and doctors. I get six to eight hours of restful sleep nearly every night. The lesson is that if you want CPAP to work for you, you may have to work for it.

I own several sizes and shapes of masks, acquired during months of trial and error—mostly error—trying to get a night's sleep. No matter what mask I was given or how carefully it was adjusted I would wake up in the middle of the night with the mask off my face. It was a victory to get one or two hours of sleep. The masks that work are ones that I have adapted with advice from a technical expert; my standby is an innovative mask from one manufacturer held in place by innovative headgear from another. My alternate is held in position by a considerable amount of double-sided Velcro tape.

The sleep laboratory used a very conservative, time-consuming protocol to evaluate my response to CPAP. As a result they couldn't get to a pressure high enough to control my sleep breathing problems during the night and it seems that the prescribed pressure wasn't high enough to suppress all apneas and hypopneas. So the prescription was probably too low. I did not understand enough about the reports to understand or question them and seek better treatment.

The home care company, in applying the prescription, used a small pressure measurement device that was only accurate to plus-or-minus two centimeters; thus the pressure applied was lower than the pressure the laboratory had recommended and the doctor had prescribed.

I have heard from others that follow-up care can be poor, so unless your caregivers are determined to take the initiative and make sure you are benefiting from optimal treatment, you may need to be responsible for your own follow-up.—J.H.

How to overcome specific problems

On the average, about 75 percent of patients treated with nasal CPAP use their machine for a long time. We will explore some of the problems that discourage patients and lead them to stop using the device, and we will review some methods to overcome these problems and make the most effective use of the therapy. Ongoing technical and medical education from qualified personnel (and sources like this book), emotional and social support from family and friends, and interaction with other patients can significantly increase the success rate. If you are prepared to get involved in your care, you increase your chances for health and happiness.

Basic setup of CPAP

The details of applying your CPAP mask and operating your machine will vary depending on the manufacturer. Observe all instructions about connecting the unit to your household current. Consider having a ground fault interrupter installed to protect the circuits in your bedroom, and the use of a surge protector. In use, CPAP units consume from 25 to 75 watts depending on the efficiency, design, and age of the unit, the type and length of tubing, and the cleanliness of the filter. If the unit is allowed to run without being worn by the patient, it will use more electricity as it puts out a maximum of effort to reach the set pressure. Thus, in normal use, the CPAP will draw about as much electricity as a light bulb.

Place the unit where it will not create a hazard in the bedroom. Be sure that the air intake is not blocked and that the unit is close enough to the bed so that there is plenty of slack in the hose. In the morning clean your mask with mild detergent, rinse it, and attach it to the blower to dry. Wash the hose once a week and attach to the blower to dry. If you are sensitive to perfumes or dyes, you may want to use a detergent without additives. Keeping filters clean is important. Follow the manufacturer's instructions. In general, you should wash reusable filters weekly and replace disposable ones monthly. You may keep a notebook or place a label on the base of the CPAP and note the dates you clean or change the filter.

Battery standby power at home

Most people probably do not need to have a standby battery at home in the event of a power failure. A power failure would mean only the loss of CPAP benefits for that night. However, if you are very uncomfortable when you miss a night of treatment, you might consider a battery backup or an uninterruptable power supply.

Mask performance

Even a minor problem can keep you from wearing the CPAP mask, because it's uncomfortable or ineffective. Most issues are easy to resolve, although careful trial and error may be necessary to solve your specific problem.

Mask types

Four major categories of masks are available, with different styles in each category.

Nasal mask

The most widely used is the *nasal mask*, a triangular plastic mask with a border of pliable material. It covers the nose and forms a seal against the skin. One manufacturer makes 'bubble' nasal masks with an additional, outer shell of pliable material to form a second air seal.

Nasal puffs

A second type is the *nasal cannulae*, which is a device to hold small tubes in or against the opening of each nostril, forming a seal. This type of device, not really a mask, is called Adam circuit, nasal puffs, nasal seal, or prongs.

Full face mask

The third type, the *full face mask,* covers both the nose and mouth. Rarely used, these masks are applied when a patient has been unable to use the other types of mask. The full face mask, developed for hospital use with monitoring and alarms to alert the staff of problems, poses certain hazards. If the machine fails, the patient can't breathe as easily as with a nasal mask and may choke on aspirated matter. If you need such a mask, your doctor will instruct you carefully in its use.

Custom masks

Finally, a number of suppliers make custom-molded masks if none of the manufactured models provides sufficient comfort and adequate seal. (See Sources of custom masks on page 123, and for further information and evaluations of masks refer to the booklet by Bud Blitzer, listed in the Bibliography on page 149.)

Some patients may keep two or more types or models of masks. If a mask breaks or proves uncomfortable, it is simple to use the other one until a replacement mask is obtained. Sometimes minor skin irritations or pimples can make a favorite mask uncomfortable, and having a different model gives the affected area a chance to rest and heal. For example, you might prefer the prongs but if an irritation or sensitivity develops in your nostril where the puffs rest, you could switch to a nasal face mask.

Headgear and adjustments

Equally important is the headgear that holds the mask on the face. The headgear should be comfortable, easy to put on, and easy to adjust. Once adjusted, it should be possible to remove the mask with the least possible need for readjustment. Some headgear allows the mask to be removed by disconnecting a single strap, leaving the adjustments unchanged. It may prove useful to mix and match headgear and masks, even from different manufacturers, so a comfortable fit and good seal can be established reliably and easily.

Comfort—part of good treatment

Each manufacturer develops variations on mask types, so there are many similar models of mask. In addition, each model may be made in different sizes. Each manufacturer may offer more than one type of harness or headgear with different features such as ease of wearing and taking off and stability in use. Nearly all masks and hoses use the same standard fitting types, thus they can be used interchangeably. With the large variety of masks and harnesses available, most patients should find one suitable. Unfortunately, the process may require trial and error until you achieve a suitable fit.

Physical discomfort from the mask and headgear can limit the utility of the CPAP device. If the mask is too tight, not only is it uncomfortable, but it can cause your eyes to swell and may lead to misalignment of your teeth. Pressure sores may develop across the bridge of your nose or elsewhere. People have experienced headaches and neck aches from pressure of the headgear on a sensitive part of the head. Your home care company or the technician or physician who prescribed or dispensed your equipment should be available to help you with the adjustments necessary to insure a correct comfortable fit. Even if the mask fits perfectly, you may find that it becomes more bothersome as time goes by and you should ask for help to improve and adjust the fit.

Mask leaks

The goal for nasal CPAP masks is to apply a good seal without undue pressure on the face or nose. If you have a mustache it is best to shave it or use the prongs type of mask. Some small leaks are probably inevitable, as you turn in your sleep or as the straps relax over the night. Most CPAP machines automatically increase flow to overcome a small leak. If there is a leak, the pressure transducer (a device that monitors the pressure delivered by CPAP) senses the drop in pressure. It calls for the blower to increase the flow of air, compensating for the leak (See Cautions on hose-length and type).

Noise

The newer models of most machines are very quiet, but they disturb some patients. While it is rare, some bed partners find the noise of a CPAP machine more disturbing than the snoring. However, the constant whisper-like drone of the blower producing pressurized air is barely audible and usually preferable to the noise of the snorer.

If you or your roommate find the normal noise of the machine unpleasant, you can isolate the unit from your sleeping area. Be careful not to restrict air intake or to prevent the unit from dissipating heat from the motor. Depending on the layout of your home, you may be able to place the head of your bed against a hallway wall, run the hose through a hole in the wall, and put the unit completely outside the room. (See cautions on hoses, below.)

If your CPAP machine has become noisier, or sounds different than when it was new, there may be a mechanical problem. Check to see that nothing is blocking the air intake, and that the filters are clean.

Sometimes a troublesome noise comes from the exhaust valve or outlet that draws off the air you exhale. Some valves make noise—and won't properly exhaust the used air—if they aren't installed correctly. If one of the ports built into the mask for administration of oxygen is open, there may be a loss of pressure as well as noise. If you have questions about your mask, refer to the instructions or ask your home care provider. Some older mask models have a noisy moving valve with a diaphragm that pops up and down with each breath. Much quieter alternatives should be substituted for these older valves.

Cautions on hose-length and type

In some devices the control circuits assume that the hose is six feet; the use of a longer hose could reduce the effectiveness of the leak-compensation system. Before extending the hose, check the instructions for your machine, ask the home care provider, or call the manufacturer. Be careful not to extend the air hose beyond the manufacturer's recommendations, and always use hose material approved by the manufacturer. The hose should be smooth bore or "laminar-flow tubing" and not internally corrugated. If you extend the hose too far or use the wrong kind of tubing, you may change the effective pressure reaching your mask, and your apneas may not be properly controlled.

CPAP pressure

The amount of pressure needed to keep your upper airway from obstructing has been determined by a careful review of your sleep, monitored and recorded at home or in the sleep laboratory, and analyzed by a technician and/ or physician. Some factors could change your ideal pressure. Changes in your health and physical condition could change the ideal pressure. For instance, if you lose weight, a lower pressure may be required, while a weight gain may require a higher pressure. If you drink alcohol or take medication that causes the upper airway muscles to relax, you might require a higher pressure to avoid apneas. Allergies, the flu, or a cold could make it less comfortable to wear the mask and interfere with your breathing, thus requiring an increase in pressure (in addition to the usual pressure used in treating your symptoms).

Adjusting pressure

Perhaps within a few years more sophisticated CPAP devices will automatically measure your response with each breath and adjust to the ideal pressure. In the meantime, consult with your technician or physician if you suspect that your pressure requirement may have changed.

You may need to do a home-monitor verification of your treatment periodically, perhaps three months after your initial titration (the determination and prescription of the effective pressure for you in an overnight test), and thereafter annually.

Assure yourself that the prescription determined by your doctor or the sleep laboratory is professionally applied and verified. Your unit should be calibrated and checked using a water manometer (the standard laboratory method, accurate to plus or minus 0.25 cm.) or an electronic pressure meter (meters should be accurate to plus or minus 0.3-0.5 cm.). Other types of measuring device can be less accurate and thus indicate the wrong pressure for your machine.

Some technical and medical personnel may be casual about setting pressures and believe that a pressure is correct if within two centimeters of the prescribed pressure. However, because the apnea response to pressure can be sensitive, precision in setting the pressure is required. The CPAP device should be set to within one-half cm. pressure of that prescribed. Because there are so many variables, such as the type and length of hose, the type of mask, and possible leaks, the best procedure is to turn on the CPAP and wear the mask, connected by tubing to the meter, as was done in the laboratory, while the pressure is adjusted and checked in your home. Since the laboratory measures the pressure at the mask when calibrating, measuring the pressure at the mask eliminates a possible source of error.

If you feel uncomfortable or think the unit is not giving you the relief you expect, ask your technician or physician to review the situation and make adjustments. Some CPAP units can be adjusted by the turn of a knob or screw, but you should resist the temptation to do it yourself. Some newer CPAP models that have electronic controls can only be set by the laboratory or a technician using external controls and measuring devices.

While patients should actively participate in treatments, they should not attempt to tailor their own treatment without the advice of medical or technical specialists. Some people may be tempted to use a CPAP device without any sleep laboratory calibration. This is not a good idea for several reasons and is unlikely to work as well as collaborating with your physician and the sleep disorders center or home care provider. A CPAP machine and its pressure setting requires a prescription as does a medication that you receive from the pharmacist. As it would be dangerous to increase or decrease medication prescribed by your doctor, changing a CPAP prescription also involves risk. Setting the pressure higher than needed to correct the obstructive apneas exposes you to unnecessary pressure and possible injury. Rarely an excessive pressure can actually promote apneas. Setting the pressure too low allows apneas to occur. Your level of daytime sleepiness alone is not sensitive enough to determine if the pressure setting is correct. Only home or laboratory monitoring can provide information for a skilled physician or technician to use to make that assessment, taking into account your feelings and observations.

In a fully equipped laboratory or with a home monitoring recorder, several kinds of data must be collected, correlated, and interpreted. The correct interpretation of sleep stages and quality requires training and expertise. The sleeper is unable to observe himself during sleep. While the patient receives a lot of information about the quality of daily life, and thus plays a critical role in evaluating treatment, casual observation cannot replace the evaluation of sleep by a technician or physician. To someone with SAS, one or two hours of sleep can feel wonderful, but to achieve a better, full night of sleep requires a precise setting of CPAP pressure. The sleep-deprived person may not always recognize the lack of competence and alertness that sleep deprivation causes. Finally, because untreated SAS can have such serious effects—it can be a killer—every available tool should be used to treat it fully and completely.

Air

Temperature

The CPAP unit may warm slightly the air passing through because the motor generates heat. If the air is noticeably warmer than the room temperature, make sure that the intake to the CPAP is not blocked and that the filter is clean. If you enjoy sleeping in a cool bedroom, but find the flow of air too cold for comfort, you can pre-warm the air with a heat-absorbing device. Simply get another length of hose (the standard length is six feet/two meters) and a suitable connector, for a total of 12 feet/four meters of air tubing. Lead the tubing under your blankets, and your body heat will warm the air.

Check the manufacturer's recommendations for acceptable hose length. If you change the hose length, the capability of the CPAP unit to maintain the prescribed pressure will be compromised. However, depending on the responsiveness of the particular CPAP unit and your own needs, a longer hose may be acceptable. Check with your physician and home-care provider. If you change the length of the air hose, check the pressure delivered at the mask. A pressure drop of about 0.5 cm of pressure may be caused by adding a six-foot/two meter hose to the system. Bends and twists in the hose can reduce the effective pressure.

Air humidity

Another frequent problem is nasal dryness and irritation from the flow of air into your nose. This problem is difficult to control. Using a saline nasal spray (available at a pharmacy) before bedtime may help. Keep the room humidity high. Some CPAP units can be attached to humidifiers. A variety of units, including heated humidifiers, is available. If you have a BiPAP unit, be sure that you use a specifically adapted humidifier. If you use an attached humidifier, pay attention to the recommendations of the manufacturer about how to keep the device and water clean. One of the main risks of using humidifiers is the growth of bacteria. If the humidifier becomes contaminated, bacteria can spread into your lungs, causing a serious infection. One manufacturer offers an "artificial nose" humidification system consisting of a sponge-like material inserted in the mask to capture moisture from the exhaled breath and to release the moisture to humidify incoming fresh air. A small supply of these might be useful when travelling instead of taking a more bulky humidifier. They seem too expensive for routine daily use in place of a humidifier.

Traveling with CPAP machines

Patients often ask if they can go without using their CPAP units for a period of time such as a weekend. Patients wonder if any problem will result from failing to use the device for a few nights. Most patients will immediately resume snoring and repeated episodes of obstructive apnea if they quit using CPAP for even one night. Others will be able to sleep well enough without it for a few nights. Going away may also mean a disruption in your normal routine, such as traveling across time zones, staying up late, and consuming alcohol. The wisest choice is to take your CPAP machine with you.

Practical travel issues

Most models of current CPAP devices are small enough to be carried in your hand onto an airplane and stowed under your seat. If you have an older, heavier model and travel frequently, it may be worthwhile to buy an easily portable machine for travel. Some of the newest models are no more trouble to carry than a briefcase. Don't check it with luggage—if it gets lost, you won't sleep well, and the risks of breakage are high.

Security checks

At the security counter, you may be asked to explain what the device is. Explain that it is a medical device to aid in your sleep, and offer to open it for inspection. If it is put through an X-ray scanner, no harm will be done to the machine and the motor, electronics, and wires will be clearly visible. Explain that you will keep it with you and that the device is designed to blow and compress air as treatment for a sleep disorder.

Customs

At customs, explain that you have a device prescribed by your doctor for your personal use when you sleep. A letter from your doctor will help. Customs is interested in finding equipment that might be taxable and be sold, but the CPAP is for your personal medical use, not for resale.

Power sources for travel

Travel by train

If you are traveling by train, you can reserve a roomette or sleeper and use the electrical outlet that delivers local standard current.

Travel by airplane

Using CPAP during a long airplane flight is possible, but you may have to make special arrangements with each airline. And you will have to determine that your CPAP can make use of the aircraft electrical power supply. Some airplanes use 110 volts at 400 Hz (compared to the usual 50-60 Hz supply in domestic use). Units made by at least one manufacturer, ResCare, can adapt to the unusual electrical supplies in such aircraft and have been cleared for use by one airline. Even after establishing that the unit is appropriate to use on their aircraft, the airline requires the passenger to apply for prior approval (at the time of making a reservation) for each flight.

You must confirm with the CPAP manufacturer that your specific unit is capable of operating at 110V at 400 Hz, the electric supply available on passenger aircraft.

Applying to the airline

Apply to the medical services of an airline, supported by a letter from your physician, and allow time for the approval process which may have to go through the engineering department as well as the medical department. Confirm the type of electrical power available.

- Apply for approval and assistance in using the CPAP during flight.
- Include a doctor's letter.
- Ask to be seated near a power outlet.
- Include information from the CPAP manufacturer including electrical requirements for voltage and frequency. The unit label and/or the documentation from the manufacturer should read 110-240V, 50-400 Hz.
- Confirm that your unit has the standard American plug and that this type of plug will fit the power outlet; or arrange to get an adapter (the physical connector, not electrical conversion) between your unit's plug and the power outlet.
- Find out if you will need to supply an electrical extension cord.

At flight time

- Bring a copy of your doctor's letter stating the need for CPAP.
- Explain to the crew the reason for your using CPAP and show them the documents from your doctor and the CPAP manufacturer and approvals from the airline.
- Show the crew the document(s) and/or unit label stating that the unit will operate at 400 Hz, 110 volts.

Foreign travel

If you are traveling overseas, get information about the places you are going and consider renting equipment suited to the local power supply.

Some CPAP devices have switchable power supplies and can use more than one electrical supply system. If so, on the back of the machine there will be a switch for selecting 220-,110-, or 12-volt settings. If your machine does not have a switchable power supply, then you can purchase a transformer to change the voltage to the correct one for use with your machine.

In a country such as Italy, you would set the switch to 220V, but you would still require an adapter to allow you to plug the machine into an electrical outlet. You should pack adapter plugs for your machine to plug into, then plug into the electrical socket (for example, foreign travel outlet adapters, Radio Shack part number 273-1405B, $8.95). Buy them before you leave—these adapters are extremely difficult to locate in foreign countries and you have better things to do on your trip. Some machines need to have the fuse changed if the electrical voltage is changed. Check the instruction booklet or contact the manufacturer. For some power supplies, you may need to purchase the appropriate electrical converter from the manufacturer. For each of these modifications or adaptations, it's a good idea to talk to the manufacturer or your home care company before embarking on a trip.

Camping

Although you won't be able to go on long hiking trips in the wilderness, CPAP treatment can go with you on camping or boating trips. It is possible to find camping sites close to a road or accessible by vehicle and thus enjoy camping and a good night's sleep. You will need to bring a battery as well as the CPAP unit and accessories. One manufacturer's representative made it possible for a 12-year-old to go on a Boy Scout camping trip by outfitting him with the appropriate battery.

For travel by car or camper, consider getting a special battery for the CPAP rather than risk draining or ruining the vehicle battery. The best choice is a deep-cycle battery made for marine or recreational vehicle use, perhaps a gel filled rather than liquid filled to avoid the risk of spills. Such batteries withstand longer use and heavy discharges, whereas ordinary batteries can be ruined by a deep discharge. To recharge this type of deep-cycle battery using the car or truck alternator may require a modification of the charging system. Depending on the type of CPAP unit and the pressure setting, you can expect to get from one to several nights of use from a deep-cycle battery depending on its size and amp-hour rating. Since a CPAP device requires from one to two amperes at most, it will use eight to 16 ampere hours each night. You can make effective use of about one-half of the rated ampere hours in a deep-cycle battery. A 30 to 40 amp-hour battery might be adequate for two nights of camping, based on information supplied by Respironics. Such batteries cost about $50-100 and weigh about 20 pounds; manufacturers include Gould, Surette, Rolls, and Atlantic. For specific examples showing the combined effects of CPAP pressure requirements, equipment electrical requirements, and battery capacity (See Nights of CPAP usage on battery). However, you should get specific information from your CPAP manufacturer and the battery manufacturer;

and before going on a trip, test your own combination of CPAP unit, pressure required, and battery capacity while you are still at home..

Table 1: Nights of CPAP usage on battery

CPAP pressure setting in cm. water	Current drawn in amps	Energy used in 8 hours (amp-hours)[a]	Nights or hours of use for a new, 60 amp-hour battery [b]	Nights or hours of use for a 30 amp-hour battery [c]
standby	0.5	4	7	3
5	1.5	12	2	1
10	2.5	20	1	6 hours
15	3.5	28	1	4 hours
20	4.5	36	6 hours	3 hours

a. The example assumes the use of a 12 to 24 volt converter (this CPAP unit runs on 24 volts). A 24-volt battery supply with the same CPAP unit and the appropriate adapter would run for 2.5 times longer in each case. This table is based on information supplied by ResCare; other manufacturers' equipment and other adapters may give different results depending on the current drawn by the specific unit and adapter.

b. About half of the rated ampere-hours can be drawn from a new, fully-charged battery, thus the battery would provide 30 amp-hours.

c. An older battery may only deliver about half of the original rating, or 30 hours in the case of a rated 60 amp-hour battery, of which only about half could be reliably used.

Medical problems of CPAP use

Caused by flow and pressure

The most common medical problems related to CPAP arise from the increased flow and pressure of air in the upper airway or from the mask against the face. If you recognize any of the following symptoms, report them to your doctor.

Drying of the upper airway

Drying of the upper airway from the increased flow of air is a typical problem, but worse in patients who sleep with their mouths open since a greater flow of air goes through the upper airway. The tissues that line the breathing passages warm and humidify air entering your lungs. When they are dry, they become irritated, crusty, and can bleed. The use of a humidifier and saline nose drops are partial solutions to this problem. Patients who have chronic nasal problems such as hay fever or rhinitis may require additional treatment to prevent nasal irritation from CPAP. For the short-term management of nasal congestion from a cold, a few days' use of a decongestant nasal spray (e.g., Afrin) is acceptable, with your doctor's approval. For longer term management of hay fever or chronic rhinitis, a local nasal spray such as cromolyn sodium (Nasalcrom) or topical cortisone preparation may help.

Cautions with cold and allergy medications

Oral medications for runny nose or colds (obtainable over the counter) usually contain antihistamines and decongestants. Sleep apnea patients should use these medications cautiously, if at all. Antihistamines can worsen daytime sleepiness; oral decongestants may lead to insomnia. Discuss any medication (even nonprescription) with your doctor before taking it. A small percentage of patients will find nasal and upper airway problems so troublesome that they will be unable to continue nasal CPAP use.

Sinus problems and nosebleeds

CPAP pressure exerted on the nasal sinuses can lead to congestion and occasionally to infection. Notify your doctor if you have sinus pain or headache, excessive, malodorous, or colored nasal discharge, a cough, or a fever.

Rarely, patients have had nosebleeds from nasal CPAP. Saline nose drops or sprays and humidification are good measures to combat nosebleeds. A nosebleed is a potentially serious problem, so notify your doctor if one happens.

Irritation of the skin or eyes

Irritation of the skin where the mask is applied is common. It can occur from the pressure of the mask against the skin (especially in places such as the bridge of the nose, where a bone is directly beneath the skin), skin occlusion by the mask, or an allergy to the mask material. Keeping your skin clean and washing your mask daily are important. The mask may need to be adjusted for fit or replaced by another type or size mask. Alert your doctor or therapist to these problems—usually, he or she will be able to find a solution.

Swelling around the eyes ('baggy eyes') in the morning may indicate a too tight mask. Irritation of the eyes or matter in your eyes in the morning often means an air leak is blowing air into your eyes during the night.

Other problems and effects from CPAP treatment

Unusual problems from nasal CPAP are changes in teeth alignment (primarily the upper front teeth), ear aches or infections, and stomach bloating from swallowing air. Patients without front teeth may need dentures, since some CPAP masks rely upon the front teeth as a point of support.

Finally, CPAP can strongly affect sleep. Most of the influence will be favorable, as your breathing is restored to normal. Occasionally, patients will experience sleepwalking during the first several nights of CPAP therapy. Sleepwalking is a manifestation of a rebound of deep sleep. Although it is rare and does not usually continue for more than a few days, you should report it to your doctor.

New complications will certainly be reported as more and more patients use CPAP therapy. Still, more than 300,000 patients have greatly benefited from this device, most of them safely, with no serious problems reported. Remember that CPAP is a medical device dispensed by prescription and used under the supervision of your physician. Users of CPAP should promptly report any unusual symptoms to their doctors.

Hospitalization with CPAP

Even in the hospital, you will sleep better and recover faster if you keep using CPAP. Discuss the fact that you have sleep apnea with your referring physician and/or the admitting physician and make arrangements to use your CPAP unit in the hospital so that you will be able to get the rest you need for recovery. In some hospitals, regular admitting procedures may not allow you to bring your own device. In such a case, the respiratory therapy department of the hospital should provide you with a CPAP unit for use during your hospitalization. You can and should, however, bring your own mask and headgear. Your primary-care physician can alert your other doctors and specialists about your needs as a sleep apnea patient. Bring a letter from your doctor with you to the hospital.

In hospitals which allow use of your personal machine, you may still need to get approval from the biomedical department. They will want to ascertain that the equipment meets hospital electrical standards, including the plug. These requirements may be satisfied if you have a double-insulated equipment (two-prong plug) or a grounded electrical system (three-prong plug). Ask about such requirements before you go to the hospital. Bring a copy of Appendix B on page 125 for information if you are going to be admitted to the hospital for any reason as well as to have surgery or any procedure that involves anesthesia, muscle relaxants, or tranquillizers during surgery, dental, or medical procedures.

Maintenance of CPAP units

Masks

Masks should be replaced if they become stiff, cracked, or broken, or don't seal well. Don't try to repair them with tape or glue.

Hoses

Hoses should be checked for leaks monthly. Turn on the machine, block the open end of the hose, and run your hands over the length of the hose and the connectors and feel for leaks.

Preventing infections

To prevent possible infection, the hose, humidifier, and mask should be kept clean and disinfected once or twice a week, or after any infection such as a cold. Avoid the use of alcohol or bleach, which may degrade the plastics in the equipment. You may use vinegar or quaternary ammonia.

Disassemble the equipment. Wash and scrub all surfaces in a warm solution of tap water and detergent.

Rinse off all detergent with tap water.

Vinegar

Prepare a solution of one part white vinegar to three parts distilled water. For example, 16 ounces vinegar to 48 ounces of distilled water.

Soak the equipment in the solution for one hour. (Discard the solution after use.)

Rinse with tap water and drain dry. (Do not wipe the equipment.)

Quaternary ammonium

Quaternary ammonium compunds (such as Control III), which may be more economical than vinegar, can be purchased through a home care company or a drugstore. Don't exceed the recommended times to avoid the possibility of degrading the plastics. Be sure to rinse well, drain dry, or attach to the blower to dry.

How to deal with insurance companies

The most important things to find out

Do you have coverage for:

- sleep evaluation;
- CPAP titration;
- CPAP equipment (DME, or durable medical equipment).

Do you have to do anything else such as obtain prior approval, before you get the coverage?

Follow these steps:

How your insurance company or health plan (if you have one) will handle your CPAP needs is unpredictable. For a long time, most insurers refused to recognize and cover the costs of diagnosis or outpatient treatment with CPAP. Check with your insurer before the laboratory test and, if CPAP is ordered, before the machine is delivered, to be sure that they will cover the costs adequately. Frequently, a letter from your doctor will be required. Many insurers will rent the machine for one to three months before purchasing it. If the patient is unable to tolerate CPAP, it is usually apparent within the first few months, so this policy is reasonable.

Insurance policies that include health care for sleep disorders including SAS can neither be explained nor described simply or comprehensively. The local offices of each organization may have different guidelines and practices. Even national, federal programs such as Medicare, Medicaid, and Social Security are administered differently in each region of the country. Rational arguments, economic considerations, and the latest scientific and medical understanding may have little impact on the coverage and reimbursement policies. As a result, patients may not receive the treatment they need. But untreated SAS can lead to accidents, death, or complications resulting in much costlier medical treatments and insurance payments. Falling asleep while driving could result in serious injuries, requiring expensive hospitalization and rehabilitation—which the insurer *would* cover. The cost of treatment for the medical and psychological treatments for the severe, chronic complaints that may be the results of untreated SAS such as high blood pressure, heart disease, stroke, or depression may be automatically covered by many insurance plans, yet these costs may far exceed the relatively modest costs of treating an underlying sleep disorder, thus saving money in the long run.

Administrators may not even be familiar with the term, sleep apnea syndrome, let alone specific appropriate ways to evaluate disability caused by a sleep disorder. However, bureaucratic obstacles to disability payments for those not restored to health may be eroding. Recently, the application of one patient for Social Security assistance was rejected because he was able to lift a 10-pound object and carry it 20 feet. However, on appeal, an administrative law judge for Social Security has ruled in this case that SAS and related illnesses, such as restless leg syndrome and depression, can together render a person eligible for long term disability.

In dealing with insurance agents, you must be extremely patient, persistent, calm, and well organized. A spouse or family member might undertake this job, since the person suffering from untreated SAS may not have the stamina and good humor necessary to deal with bureaucracies. Remember, everyone is doing their job, so your task is to understand their job and work within the system(s). Always introduce yourself and ask the name and job title of the person you are speaking with. When someone says, "No," ask in your most calm and pleasant voice, "Why?" And listen carefully, because within the regulation that prompts the "No," is a reason that might justify a "Yes." Take dated notes on every conversation, write letters that confirm even obvious points of agreement, and go back for additional clarification. Help administrators to do their jobs by giving them information you have learned from another agency (if it is not confidential), and find reasons to enable them to do their jobs by helping you. The patient may be the one common point of contact among all the caregivers and the insurer, so the patient (or your representative) must be prepared to coordinate the efforts of all. While your personal physician can be a great and indispensable helper and resource, you must do much of the research and negotiations.

If you are completely frustrated and feel like crying, do it! Sometimes admitting how much you care and how painful the frustration is can move the most hardheaded administrator to take pity and explain which exceptions to the rules might be used in your favor. Finally, no matter how angry or frustrated you get, never forget to say "Please" and "Thank you," because you are dealing with basically decent people who want to help people like you, and they may be just as angry or frustrated with the system.

If you have serious health and performance problems due to SAS, and you encounter unusually difficult problems getting coverage for your treatment, discuss with your doctor the possibility of renting equipment for a trial period or while you negotiate insurance payments. Later you may purchase the needed equipment. If you can afford the cost of a laboratory or home study ($800 to $1,200 for a diagnostic study and $800 to $1,200 for titrating the CPAP prescription), and pay $1,000 to $1,200 for a CPAP device, or rental fees of about $100 per month, this may be one of the best investments you have ever made. Your increased earning power alone, if your treatment is effective, could justify the cost. Of course, these figures do not include the specialists and tests that may be required to rule out other diseases or complications.

Fortunately, more and more health maintenance organizations and insurers are recognizing the value of CPAP therapy as an economic proposition—it may cost less to treat SAS than the injuries and illness that can result from untreated SAS.

Chapter 9

What else can you do?

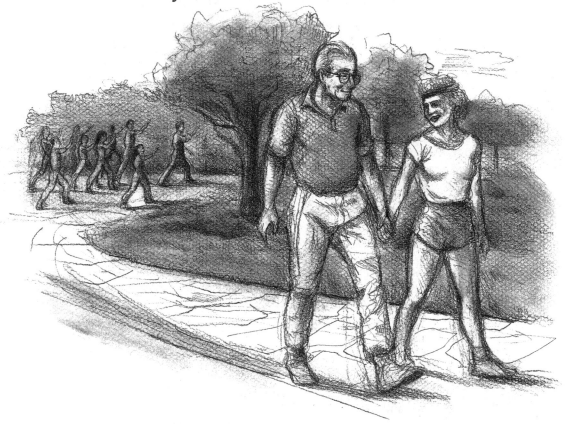

Getting better sleep can be part of a general renewal of one's life and be aided by losing weight through diet and exercise.

Figure 9.1

Learning the hard way

What I didn't know was hurting me. For many years I smoked a pipe, cigarettes, and cigars. In the evening, to relax and sleep better, I would have whiskey. I never realized that I was making my snoring worse and creating conditions for SAS.

Over the years I had gained a lot of weight. As an adolescent I had been thin and weak, so I was pleased to be larger and more substantial. I didn't see the connection between my daytime fatigue and my sleep breathing, nor did I imagine that the quality of my sleep could be affected by my weight and how much I ate.

To reduce an annoying post-nasal drip and make it easier to sleep, I used an over-the-counter drug. During treatment for SAS I always noted this drug on my questionnaire for my doctors and sleep laboratories. No one ever questioned the wisdom of using it. Only when a friend who is a nurse told me that this drug was not good to take if I had a sleep disorder—since it is a stimulant— did I realize what I was doing to myself. Stopping this medication earned me an extra hour or two of sleep each night.—J.H.

What you can do

Clean up your act—sleep hygiene

Many SAS patients suffer from poor sleep because of habits they have developed around their sleep environment and timing. Although sleep is a naturally occurring phenomenon, it can easily be subverted. The harder one tries to sleep, the less likely sleep is to come.

Sleep doctors often talk about sleep hygiene. They are referring to simple, non-medicinal practices designed to reinforce the normal sleep drive that we all possess. To treat many sleep disorders, sleep hygiene remains the only feasible approach. Many of sleep hygiene principles aid the chronically poor sleeper (the insomniac), but they can improve any patient's sleep, including the person with SAS. Here are some important do's and don'ts:

- Sleep in a comfortable, quiet, dark, and safe room you use exclusively for sleeping. The room's temperature should suit your preference but be slightly cool (around 70 degrees).

- Your bedtime should be somewhat flexible, reflecting the needs of the day. However, waking time should be absolutely unchanging. The best way to establish and maintain good sleep is to create a ritual of awakening in the morning at the same time. This schedule reinforces the body's internal time-keeper, which promotes wakefulness beginning around sunrise.

- Remove from the bedroom external influences such as the television set. Television is much too stimulating for bedtime.

- Following a regular exercise routine in the daytime promotes good sleep if it occurs at the right time of day. Avoid late-evening exercise which is too invigorating. For the beneficial effects of exercise on sleep to occur, you need time to wind down and let the body relax. Vigorous exercise (such as running marathons) increases deep sleep (stages 3 and 4).

- If you are prone to insomnia, read for a few minutes before turning out the light. If you find yourself unable to get to sleep within a reasonable amount of time, and are getting frustrated lying in bed, then get out of bed, go into another room, and read or do some other restful activity. Once you begin to feel sleepy again you should return to bed.

- Eating a light snack or taking a warm bath an hour or so before bed helps many people sleep.

- Caffeine, even limited to the morning hours, and alcohol, especially consumed in the evening, are bad influences. If you are having any kind of sleep problem, you should eliminate these drugs as well as cigarette smoking. Some prescription medications and over-the-counter remedies also affect sleep. If you take any medication, discuss its potential effects on sleep with your doctor.

These simple suggestions are based on the principle that our internal clocks control sleep as well as on observations of what effectively treats common sleep problems. For the apnea patient, however, these nonspecific approaches are not sufficient, since a specific problem occurs with breathing during sleep. If this fundamental disturbance is not corrected, then other approaches will be of limited benefit. Thus sleep hygiene should be used in addition to one or more treatments for apnea. We discussed CPAP therapy in Chapter 7. Now we will discuss upper airway surgery, weight loss, medications, and other measures for the management of sleep apnea.

Weight loss

A close relationship between obesity and snoring has been noted for centuries. At least 50 percent of patients with SAS are overweight, some greatly but many just slightly. Weight reduction benefits the majority of patients. Modest weight reductions are often enough to improve the quality of sleep in apnea patients. A weight loss of 15 to 20 pounds may be all that is needed. The reasons are not clear. The most straightforward explanation is that when excess fat is lost from the neck area and the internal tissues of the upper airway, the airway for breathing increases in size. Muscle tension in the upper airway may also improve during weight loss, for unknown reasons.

It is unfortunate that losing weight is so difficult because it is undeniably the best therapy for sleep apnea when it is successful and it has many other positive health benefits. Sleep-deprived patients have poor appetite control and even rely on food as a stimulant. Consequently, weight loss is particularly difficult. For many patients, the restoration of normal sleep with CPAP will then enable them to lose weight. In addition, a referral from your doctor to a nutritionist or a weight loss clinic should be considered.

Monitoring treatment progress

Since weight loss may change the CPAP pressure needed to control your apneas, you may find it helpful to chart your weight, keep a sleep log, and carefully monitor your daytime status. You should also ask your physician to periodically review your treatment perhaps using a home monitoring or sleep lab evaluation.

Other medical or surgical possibilities

Can surgery cure sleep apnea?

Some people were born to snore. Their families produced heroic snorers. Some of these snorers have inherited facial and throat structures that promote snoring. Others may have other anatomic problems. Surgery may be the best solution for certain of these patients. The main objective of surgery on the upper airway is to enlarge the air passage during sleep so that obstruction and apnea are prevented. Potential sites for surgical therapy are the nose, the jaw, the tongue, and the throat.

Surgical aproaches

The nose

Some causes of nasal obstruction can be treated with medication, but others require surgery. Nasal obstructions can cause snoring. To overcome the resistance to the flow of air, greater suction pressure is needed to draw air in past the obstruction. This pressure pulls the flexible tissues in the back of the throat closer together, causing vibration and noise. The precise cause of nasal obstruction is not important—any obstruction increases the chances of snoring, which disturbs sleep. Removing the obstruction to improve the flow of air may eliminate snoring and apnea and improve the quality of sleep. Derek Lipman, M.D., an ear-nose-throat (ENT) specialist explains several surgical options in his useful book, *Stop Your Husband From Snoring.*

Some patients' sleep apnea can be improved or cured by correcting deformities of the nasal passage. One common deformity corrected surgically is the deviated nasal septum, the tissue that runs down the middle of the inside of the nose and separates the left and right nasal passages. If it is not directly in the middle but shifted to one side, it is deviated, which may make breathing through the smaller nostril difficult. Often, surgery on the nose to correct the septal deviation will be coupled with surgical reduction of the nasal turbinates, the fleshy outgrowths in the nose that increase its surface area.

Tracheostomy

Surgery has often been used to treat the anatomic abnormalities of sleep apnea victims. In the 1970s, the first procedure used to treat severe sleep apnea was *tracheostomy.* This surgical procedure creates a permanent hole ("stoma") in the neck through which one breathes at night. A small cylindrical tube passes from the skin to the windpipe. One end opens into the windpipe and the other can be opened to admit air.

In the day, a cap covers the end of the tube so that breathing and speech take place normally. At night the cap is removed so that breathing can occur primarily through the surgical opening. Tracheostomy is the most radical and direct way to deal with obstructing tissue in the throat, since it bypasses the region entirely. No matter how much obstruction develops in the nose and throat, a passageway is open in the neck to breathe through.

The first patients who are recognized with a new disease are often the most flagrant examples of the disease—the tip of the iceberg that is most visible. In the late 1970s and early 1980s, when tracheostomy was introduced, it successfully treated many patients severely ill with sleep apnea. Despite sometimes serious complications, the majority of these patients were truly cured. Breathing through their tracheostomies, they finally experienced restful sleep. Even today an occasional patient may require a tracheostomy if the disease is severe and other approaches fail.

The throat: UPPP (uvulopalatopharyngoplasty)

With all its potential complications, however, a tracheostomy is unacceptable to doctors and patients for the treatment of milder sleep apnea. New surgical procedures have been introduced since 1970, including a widely used operation that goes by the tongue-twisting name of *uvulopalatopharyngoplasty* (shortened to UPP, UPPP, or UP3). This surgical procedure on the uvula, the soft palate, and the pharynx (throat) removes excess tissue to enlarge the airway passage and reduce the floppiness of the airway tissues. UPPP works well to reduce snoring. More than eighty percent of patients report disappearance or marked reduction in snoring (usually, as observed by spouses). Unfortunately only about 50 to 65 percent of patients have a significant (greater than 50 percent) reduction in apneas following UPPP. Also, in one study, patients treated with UPPP had as great a chance of dying over the following eight years as patients who were not treated. In the same study, patients treated with CPAP or tracheostomy had a lower chance of dying compared to untreated patients. Based on these observations and additional clinical studies it appears that:

- Patient selection for UPPP is very important. The best results are reported for young patients who are not severely obese, who have moderate sleep apnea, and who have obstruction at the level of the soft palate.

- A follow-up sleep study is mandatory after UPPP (as well as other therapies) to determine if success was achieved.

- More studies are needed to define the role of upper airway surgery for treatment of sleep apnea (and, indeed, to define the risk of untreated sleep apnea).

Very few patients have complications resulting from the UPPP. However, the risks include nasal regurgitation, narrowing of the throat, change in voice, and as with most surgical procedures, a few deaths have been reported. Nasal regurgitation can be troublesome. When a patient is swallowing, fluid or food may flow up into the nasal cavity or out the nose because the uvula and soft palate can no longer effectively block off the nasal passage during swallowing.

The upper and lower jaw bones

The lower jaw is the site for the attachment of the muscles that pull the tongue and pharyngeal muscles forward and keep the throat open. An abnormally positioned or small jaw sets the stage for obstruction of the airway during sleep, in the lower region of the throat, behind and below the back of the tongue. Two surgical procedures seek to remedy these lower jaw abnormalities. The simpler one (genioglossus advancement with hyoid myotomy-suspension) moves a small portion of the anterior chin to advance and tighten the tongue muscles—it does not move the jaw or teeth. The more complex procedure (maxillary-mandibular advancement osteotomy) moves both the upper and lower jaw bones forward. A sequential surgical approach, starting with the simpler procedure combined with a UPPP and then progressing to the more complex procedure if apnea persists, has been advocated by Nelson Powell and others in the Stanford Sleep Disorders Center, particularly for patients with a facial skeletal deformity. These procedures are more complex than operations on the nose or pharynx since they involve the readjustment and remodeling of bone and tooth bite. However, they have been successful in correcting sleep apnea for selected patients. The more complex procedure proved very successful for patients having undergone unsuccessful UPPP, for those not cured by the simple procedure, and persons with facial skeletal deformity.

Other surgical techniques

Surgeons continue to develop novel approaches for the management of snoring and sleep apnea since no operation or medical device is ideal. Recently, for example, the use of lasers to resect portions of the base of the tongue or of the soft palate have received widespread attention. Careful selection of your surgeon and a full understanding of the risks and benefits of the operation should accompany the decision to undertake any form of surgery for sleep apnea.

Other non-surgical approaches

Some patients who only snore or have very mild sleep apnea feel that the CPAP device interferes with sleep. Nasal CPAP can usually eliminate snoring, but for a patient without sleep apnea, whose snoring may be mostly embarrassing or annoying to a bed partner, the device is too disruptive compared to the benefits. Yet undergoing upper airway surgery is considered too extreme an approach by many patients.

Medications

Because obstructive sleep apnea is found in patients with a smaller upper airway than in non-sufferers, it is not surprising that medicines have not been very successful in remedying the situation. Most of the drugs that have been tried are stimulants, either of the whole nervous system or of the breathing system. Medications include: acetazolamide, medroxyprogesterone, nicotine, strychnine, theophylline, protriptyline, almitrine, naloxone, and oxygen. In certain unique situations these drugs have proven beneficial. Acetazolamide is effective with the central form of sleep apnea. This drug and medroxyprogesterone (MPA) are stimulants of breathing. MPA appears useful in certain very obese patients with obstructive sleep apnea whose breathing is also impaired during the day. Theophylline is a drug very similar in chemical structure to caffeine and is primarily used to treat asthma by strengthening the muscles of breathing and opening up constricted lower airways. Although scientific studies have not found it to be consistently useful in obstructive sleep apnea, it continues to enjoy some popularity, particularly in Europe. A small group of patients who have SAS in relationship to heart failure can be beneficially treated with theophylline. Like its relative, caffeine, theophylline disturbs sleep, limiting its usefulness.

Protriptyline and similar drugs developed for the treatment of depression inhibit dream sleep. Since severe apneas occur during dream sleep, a decrease in dream sleep usually means that apneas decline as well. Unfortunately, the drug has many side effects that limit its use—constipation, dry mouth, and sexual dysfunction—so that it has not gained wide acceptance as a treatment for SAS.

Finally, when SAS is a feature of an endocrine disease (hypothyroidism or acromegaly), then treatment of the underlying disease may alleviate sleep apnea.

Some medications, including all sedatives, hypnotics, and sleep-inducing medications except antihistamines, should be avoided because they may induce or worsen apnea. (See Appendix B on page 125.)

Sleep positioning

Some patients snore only when lying on their backs. Apneas are usually more frequent and severe when patients sleep on their back. One-third to one-half of patients exhibit sleep apneas only on their backs. These individuals typically are less obese and have less severe obstructions. Several devices attempt to control a sleeping person's posture and prevent or make uncomfortable the supine (back) position. The simplest consists of a pocket sewn into the back of a T-shirt or a pair of pajamas. The patient puts a ball (ranging from the size of a squash ball to a tennis ball) in the pocket. The lump pushes into his back whenever he rolls over. This variation on the princess and the pea works for some people, however patients may learn to adjust to this device and continue to sleep in a supine, snoring position. In a similar vein, audible alarms which sound when the patient rolls onto his or her back have proven useful. Straps to hinder rolling completely over are also in use. For the patient with exclusively positional apnea these devices are worth trying, especially in conjunction with weight loss. Repeat sleep studies should be performed regularly to ensure continued success.

Oral appliances

Over a dozen types of oral appliances are available for the control of snoring and sleep apnea. These devices are designed to hold the mouth open slightly, pull the lower jaw forward, move the tongue forward, or some combination of these. The theory is that snoring and apnea will be diminished if the device can lead to an increased size of the upper airway passage. It should be emphasized that most of these devices have not been subjected to the kinds of clinical studies that confirm their treatment success (as have, for example, nasal CPAP and tracheostomy). Consequently, caution must be exercised in their use. This caution does not mean that the devices are never useful. If a doctor or dentist suggests using such a device, however, they should answer the following questions to your satisfaction before you adopt it.

- How many patients with my problem (i.e., sleep apnea) have used such a device?
- Does the device completely eliminate apneas during sleep?
- What are the possible side effects of the treatment?
- How many devices has the doctor or dentist personally fitted or used?

Furthermore, if you snore but do not know if you have sleep apnea, then a sleep evaluation prior to the use of any treatment device is mandatory.

Tongue retaining device

One oral appliance that has been studied in clinical trials is the tongue retaining device (TRD). The TRD works to hold the tongue forward in the mouth so that it cannot fall into the back of the throat as the muscles relax with sleep. The TRD must be heat molded and trimmed to fit a patient individually, a procedure usually done by a specially trained dentist. This device seems to be best suited for patients that are not very obese and have strongly positional apnea.

Other dental appliances pull the lower jaw forward to increase the space in the back of the throat and may be helpful for mild apnea and snoring. The main complications from oral appliances are excessive salivation, soreness in the mouth, and change in bite.

The ideal therapy

The ideal therapy for sleep apnea should accomplish the following goals:

- eliminate all apneas and provide normal breathing during sleep
- establish restful, restorative sleep
- return daytime functioning to normal
- prevent premature death, strokes, etc. from sleep apnea
- be free of complications
- be inexpensive, readily available, and acceptable to patient and bed partner.

When weight loss is successful, this approach may be the only one that meets all of these criteria. All other modes of therapy, including CPAP and surgery, fail in one or another of these goals. Since so many personal, medical, and situational factors must be considered in each individual case, treatment selection is a matter for discussion between patient and doctor. Numerous options are available for treatment of the sleep apnea. Given the many factors, you need to discuss the alternatives with your personal physician before making a decision. Unfortunately, the choice of many treatment options indicates that no single method is uniformly effective and acceptable. But with available methods, your sleep apnea should be controllable. Whatever method is used, however, be sure to have follow-up studies and to monitor the success of the treatment on a regular basis.

The following table may be helpful as a basis for reviewing the options open to each patient.

Table 2: Comparison of therapies for sleep apnea syndrome

Treatment	Risks or complications of treatment	Apnea elimination— normal sleep breathing, good sleep, normal daytime functioning	Prevents death or other medical complications of SAS	Acceptable to patient, bed partner; cost and availability
Weight loss	Considered safe if undertaken sensibly and with medical supervision	Possible	Probable, if apnea is fully eliminated	Requires life-style adjustments, can be used together with other treatments

Table 2: Comparison of therapies for sleep apnea syndrome

Treatment	Risks or complications of treatment	Apnea elimination—normal sleep breathing, good sleep, normal daytime functioning	Prevents death or other medical complications of SAS	Acceptable to patient, bed partner; cost and availability
CPAP	Few serious medical risks. Living with CPAP involves numerous hygiene and comfort problems that can be avoided or controlled by the patient working with physician	Yes	Yes	Readily available at moderate cost, often covered by insurance. Acceptable to many patients and bed partners. Requires persistence and discipline.
Surgery on nasal passage	Risks of surgery; nasal irritation and dryness.	Success varies	Not established	Readily available at moderate cost, often covered by insurance. Acceptable to most patients and bed-partners.
Tracheostomy	Risks of surgery. Numerous problems living with tracheostomy.	Yes	Yes	Rarely used except in severe cases because CPAP provides equivalent benefits without surgery.
Surgery on jaw	Risks of surgery; prolonged recovery.	Successful in selected patients	Not established	Expensive and not widely available
Surgery on tongue	Risks of surgery; difficulty swallowing	Success varies	Not established	Only done by a small number of centers
UPPP surgery	Risks of surgery; nasal regurgitation, difficulty swallowing	Reduction in apnea index in 50-60% of patients; patient selection important	Not established	Widely available
Tongue retaining device	Tongue and gum soreness	Partial reduction, useful in selected patients	Not established	Generally available; moderate expense
Other oral devices	Tongue and gum soreness	Not known	Not established	Available

Table 2: Comparison of therapies for sleep apnea syndrome

Treatment	Risks or complications of treatment	Apnea elimination—normal sleep breathing, good sleep, normal daytime functioning	Prevents death or other medical complications of SAS	Acceptable to patient, bed partner; cost and availability
Position control	Patient may stop responding; should be retested	Some reduction in apnea and snoring in positional apnea	Not established	Combine with weight loss
Medications	Varies with each medication	Not very successful although some benefits obtained depending on situation. Good if there is an underlying thyroid condition	Not established	Varies with each medication

Chapter 10

Breathe, sleep, and live

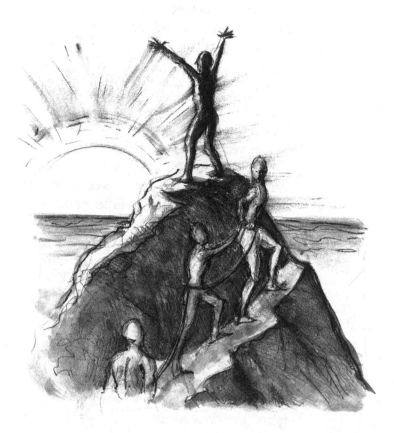

Alone and with others, there is a path to recovery

for each person with SAS.

Figure 10.1

My path to recovery

For many years I stumbled through life, unable to understand why things were going so badly. Out of my experience and advice and information from many others, I have created this path for recovery. I occasionally review these steps to monitor my own treatment.

Before I meet my doctor, I prepare a list of questions and problems and a review of my progress. If I have forgotten something or don't feel right about things, I write my doctor a note. My doctor responds by listening carefully, answering my questions, and helping me to understand the next test or treatment change. The more I understand and get involved in my own treatment, the more I appreciate my doctor's support and objective point of view—and the more I value her advice. I feel good when my doctor listens to my ideas and asks for my ideas about what might help.

Although my health plan assigns a specialist pulmonologist to follow my sleep apnea treatment, I include my internist, because sleep apnea may affect many other areas of treatment. I expect to maintain this level of attention and involvement for the rest of my life, at least whenever I have a specific sleep-related complaint. I'm still learning how to breathe while I sleep.

After successful treatment using CPAP I nevertheless continued to gain weight. This probably caused the need for a higher CPAP pressure. Later, as I recovered my energies and my life improved, I decided to lose weight by changing my eating habits. But I didn't watch my weight, thinking that after a few weeks I could see the results. As I began to lose weight, however, many old symptoms of sleep apnea syndrome crept up on me. I fell asleep while on a bus in the evening and had to fight to keep my eyes pen while working at a computer. My level of functioning in work declined as simple problems seemed too complex to untangle. My enthusiasm and energy diminished, and I shuffled the same problems from one pile to another without making any real progress. I began to feel morose and mildly depressed and then anxious, lest I be unable to carry out my plans.

I began again to keep a detailed sleep log, and remedied everything that came to mind. To combat allergies and nasal stuffiness, I replaced the air filters on the CPAP device twice a week and even bought a new air cleaner to get relief from airborne allergens. I reviewed the sleep hygiene situation, and even got to bed earlier so that I would be sleeping longer. But I still wasn't sleeping well.

Desperate and frightened, I called my doctor and demanded help, and we agreed to get an immediate sleep test. Fortunately, an opening was quickly available and I had a full study with calibration. The lowest pressure tried (which the technician assumed would be below my needs) turned out to provide excellent relief. Apparently the weight loss had reduced my pressure requirements and the old pressure may have been creating central apneas, a problem sometimes seen with excess pressure.

With the new prescription, I began sleeping well again and I experienced the renewed energy, enthusiasm, and improvement in performance in all areas of my life including work, social, emotional, and sexual. As I looked with fresh eyes at my life, I had the uncomfortable feeling that someone else had been recently in my place—a confused, incompetent, tired person pretending to be me. Here was another reminder that CPAP users must be constantly alert and involved in treatment, and that this effort can help bring about success.

The sleep test, however, raised some new questions when the doctor reviewed the results. Although the sleep apnea was fully controlled by CPAP, nevertheless the amount and type of sleep seemed unusual. Thus some other possibilities needed checking. To explain some remaining problems, I keep a daily sleep log of how well I feel, how I have slept, and variables that might affect my sleep. Keeping the log helps me see where I could improve my sleep. If I feel depressed or people around me seem critical of my performance, I pay attention to my sleep and can often figure out what can be done to improve matters. With the problem of sleep apnea syndrome finally under control, it would now be possible to resolve any remaining problems and perhaps get even better quality sleep.—J.H.

Discovering, treating, and recovering from SAS

If you suspect that you have SAS, you can play a major part in your diagnosis, treatment, and recovery process. The following steps will help you organize your efforts and remind you of key elements that may affect your progress. The main idea is to learn how to work more effectively as an informed patient to get the most out of the skills and experience that your doctor and the health care system can bring to you. Remember, if you have SAS you may not be aware of the problem. However, your spouse, family, friends, and colleagues can give you important clues and more. Before you reject expressions of criticism or concern, consider if people may be concerned or upset because you are not behaving or performing up to your normal potential.

Do you have a problem breathing during sleep?

To seek help, you must recognize that a problem exists. One of the great obstacles in the care of sleep apnea is the difficulty that the patient has in realizing that daytime symptoms may result from impaired sleep. First, carefully review the checklist of questions on page 19 in Chapter 3 and the following examples. If you have a bed partner, ask him or her to answer them with you.

If you are not sleeping well, your symptoms may be caused by sleep apnea or another sleep disorder. Many symptoms can also be caused by other medical or psychiatric problems. Therefore, even if sleep apnea is not the basis for your symptoms, they deserve attention from your doctor.

If you snore and have pauses in breathing during sleep, the reason for your daytime sleepiness and other symptoms may be sleep apnea. Snoring, especially loud nightly snoring, pauses in breathing during sleep, and excessive daytime sleepiness are the strongest indicators of sleep apnea.

Collect more information.

Keep a sleep log

Your doctor will need more information, which you can provide. You can learn much about yourself and your sleep habits by collecting information. A sleep specialist would ask you to keep a sleep log as the first order of business. A sleep log is a daily diary of your sleep maintained over a few weeks. Sleep logs are useful no matter what type of problem you have, whether sleep apnea, insomnia, or shift work. Use a small notebook or a calendar large enough to make entries for each day. A useful form that you may copy for personal use is the Sleep log form on page 131. Each morning enter the following information:

❑ What medications, caffeine, or alcohol if any, did you take during the previous day, especially in the evening?

❑ What time did you go to bed last night?

❑ What time did you turn out the lights and try to sleep?

❑ What time did you fall asleep—how long did it take you to fall asleep?

❑ How many awakenings did you have last night?

❑ How well did you sleep (on a scale of 1 to 10 scale with 10 being the best)?

❑ What other observations can you make (such as whether you snored during the night, whether you awakened with a headache, etc.)?

❑ What time did you wake up this morning?

❑ How many hours did you sleep?

If you are excessively sleepy in the daytime, you can enter additional comments on the quality of your day such as number of naps or how sleepy you felt (on a 1 to 10 scale, with 10 being uncontrollably sleepy). Pay particular attention to keeping the log over weekends and holidays, times when you are not forced to maintain a work schedule. Observations from these times often reveal much about the body's underlying rhythm of sleep. Since much of what you eat, drink, and do influences sleep, it is important to include information about these items in your log. For example, include how much caffeine (coffee, tea, or cola) and alcohol you drink and when. Since drugs, including nonprescription drugs, are another potential source of sleep disturbance, don't forget to include them. Finally, note the timing of exercise. When you first see your doctor, bring this sleep log to document your sleep problem.

Make a tape recording

Another useful technique for examining your sleep pattern is an audio recording. Often, a patient's spouse or family will make an audio recording to prove to the disbelieving patient the intensity of the snoring. Ideally, a sleep recording should last at least 90 minutes so that a full cycle of dream sleep and quiet sleep can be recorded.

Figure 10.2 Sleep log example

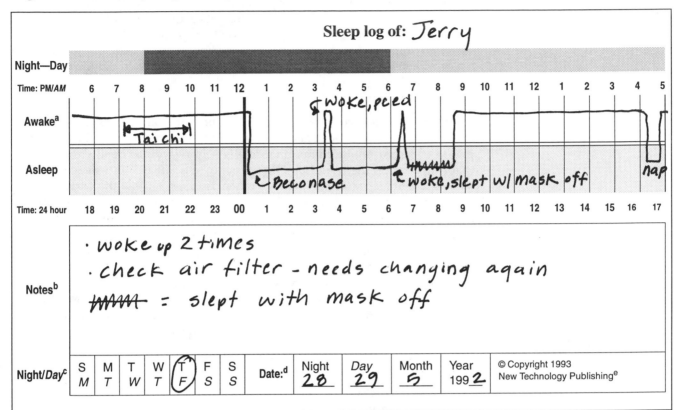

Figure 10.2 A sleep log filled out in use by a patient. The line drawn by the patient is above the horizontal divider to show awake, below to show asleep. Thus, a nap is shown by a dip, and an awakening from sleep is shown as a rise. A simple note with an arrow to mark the time can be used to show medication, exercise, symptoms, and comments. Thus the log can be used to monitor and maintain therapy.

Tape recorders with a slow speed and/or autoreverse are able to record for ninety minutes. However many cassette recorders cannot record for 90 minutes unless someone turns the tape over midway. If your bed partner will do this for you, ask whether he or she will also count the number of pauses in your breathing (if any) and measure how long they last. Count for five minutes at a time, two or three times during the recording period. A pause in breathing is easy to recognize, since the sound of snoring stops momentarily.

See your doctor.

A great physician and teacher, Francis Weld Peabody, wrote that "One of the essential qualities of the clinician is interest in humanity, for the secret of the care of the patient is in caring for the patient." Everyone needs a personal physician, a primary care doctor who provides the cornerstone of your medical care. Your personal physician cannot know all the complexities of modern medicine. Today, no physician can. But he or she can know you as a human being, your background, both personal and medical, and the details of your medical history. He or she can guide you through the maze of additional services that you need. If you have a problem that he or she cannot understand or solve, then your primary care doctor can communicate with other physicians or health-care workers. A phone call or letter from the primary physician serves as an important introduction for you to the other services that you need. Thus, an important quality of your primary-care physician is the ability to communicate—with you and other physicians—effectively. If you think you might be suffering from sleep apnea or another sleep problem, begin with your personal physician.

Another reason for working closely with your personal physician is that he or she should know you personally and be able to observe changes in you over a period of years. Another important role is helping you to deal with a disease that might fall in the territory of one or more specialists. With sleep disorders some symptoms can mimic those of other diseases. Unless the correct source (the primary disease) is identified, treating the effects or the secondary disease may provide relief, while the hidden disease continues to do damage. One example is *depression*, a serious change in mood that can be crippling unless properly treated. Even for the trained physician it is difficult to identify, diagnose, and treat depression because clinical depression may emerge in several ways: as the reaction to loss and sadness, as from the death of a loved one; by an emotional or mental disturbance; or as the outcome of a sleep disorder. Your primary-care doctor can help you to find the best path to follow, referring you to specialists and helping to coordinate their findings.

Besides your sleep log and audio recording, the answers to some other questions may be useful to your physician:

❑ Have you ever had gland (endocrine) problems? Sleep apnea has been frequently observed in patients with underactive thyroid glands, for example.

❑ Have you ever had a serious head injury, been unconscious, or in a coma?

❑ Did you have polio as a child?

❑ Did you have an infection of the brain, such as spinal meningitis or encephalitis? (Injury to the brain may be the cause of breathing difficulties during sleep).

❑ Do you have problems with your nose, such as hay fever, or other allergies, chronic sinus congestion, or nosebleeds?

❑ Has anyone in your family (including close relatives) had problems with snoring or excessive sleepiness?

Help yourself.

Before you see your doctor or undergo special tests, you can begin the process of treatment and recovery. Chapter 9 includes advice to help you control your snoring. Central to these personal efforts are weight reduction and avoidance of alcohol.

Because sleep apnea is a newly recognized condition in the medical world, not every physician has learned about the risks associated with treating sleep apnea patients. Therefore you as a patient need to take on extra responsibility for your own care. You should discuss with your doctor that drivers with severe SAS have an increased risk of crashes. Until you have been evaluated and treated, don't drive a vehicle—out of consideration for the safety of your passengers, others using the highways, and to protect yourself. Your safety and well-being during routine medical and dental procedures may depend on your speaking up and explaining the medical facts and risks of sleep apnea to your doctors and dentists. Your doctors should appreciate your contribution to managing your treatment.

Don't drop the ball

The first four steps should help you understand the root of your problem. If sleep apnea seems responsible for your symptoms, then your doctor may arrange for a sleep study and consultations with other physicians may also be necessary. Chapters 5 and 6 describe the testing procedures for sleep apnea.

While you are waiting for a diagnosis and treatment to begin, you may feel too tired or exhausted to forge ahead. You may be frustrated by a long wait to see a consultant or to have a sleep study performed. Don't be discouraged—persistence will be rewarded.

Consider treatment options, then act.

Treatment options for the sleep apnea patient range from weight loss, eliminating alcohol and certain medications, to attention to sleep hygiene. In addition, nasal CPAP is effective for the majority of patients (see Chapter 7, "The Miracle of Relief"). Surgery may be indicated for you. Chapter 9 discusses the available surgical and other approaches. Finally, only you and your doctor can decide what is right for you.

Begin recovery and evaluate your progress.

Finding a treatment is one of the steps. Then you must also begin to reestablish family and work connections. With better sleep and renewed vigor this task will be easier, but patients often need help. A support group, an advisor, or a health-care professional may be of help during these times. Support and educational groups, such as AWAKE, organized by patients and health-care professionals, provide information about therapies for SAS and the chance for patients and family members to share their specific problems, challenges, and successes on a range of issues from the technical details of treatment to how patients and their loved ones feel about the process of treatment and recovery.

Self-evaluation during and after recovery is very important. Continue to ask yourself:

❑ How do you feel and how do others see you now?

❑ Are you better or worse in areas that might be related to a sleep problem?

❏ Are any old symptoms reappearing?

❏ Do people treat you as they did when you were always tired, or does feedback tell you that your behavior and performance are that of a normal, rested and alert person?

❏ What external and internal changes and signs of progress do you observe?

Your motivation and commitment

To overcome your sleep disorder may require only a small effort or a major commitment to changes that will affect your whole life and relationships with others. Your doctor can provide treatment and technology to help you, but only you can carry out the treatment and undergo the changes. Only you can decide if the level of effort is worthwhile. You may be glad in the end, but in the beginning the mountain may seem too high to climb. Your own determination and motivation will be a major factor in your success.

Fortunately for most sufferers from SAS, treatment of sleep apnea is highly successful. And, much of the thinking about apnea is filtering down to the treatment of snoring. Chronic snorers are being evaluated seriously and can benefit from therapies developed for sleep apnea.

Your doctor, perhaps consulting with sleep specialists, endocrinologists, nutritionists, ear-nose-and-throat surgeons, and others, has a range of choices to control the severest conditions of sleep apnea patients. Dietary manipulation, nasal CPAP, upper airway surgery, and medications, used singly or more likely in combination, will control your breathing at night and let you get the sound sleep you need to function as a whole person. Education, follow-up, and support can assure successful treatment and recovery.

Chapter 11

The process of recovery

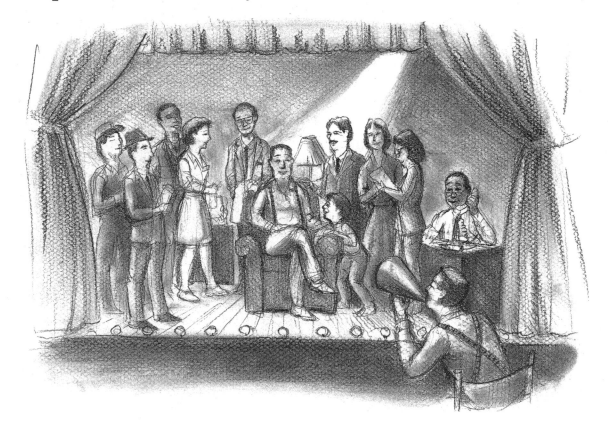

Actors in your new life—you are the director

and you play many roles

but there are many other parts to be filled.

Figure 11.1

My recovery

At one time after I had begun CPAP therapy I was getting only a couple of hours of treated sleep each night because of some technical problems. In addition to feeling fatigue and frustration, I was overwhelmed by uncertainty and depression. I had no one to talk to who understood the effects of SAS. I wondered if I could be successfully treated and become productive again. Would I be permanently incapacitated? How could I take care of myself, let alone meet my responsibilities to others? I could see no relief from the exhaustion, frustration, and uncertainty. Even the psychologist I consulted (even though he provided urgently needed support and direction) seemed critical and judgmental—why didn't I just pull myself together and do what was necessary to survive? My family and friends were also critical. Everyone had practical, sensible solutions; the problem was that I was too tired and unreliable to function or work. I was depressed and ready to jump off a bridge.

Not until I spoke with other SAS patients did I realize that many of my performance and psychological problems were directly related to SAS. A psychologist with experience treating SAS patients mentioned that many people with SAS were depressed. I could stop feeling guilty that I was tired, depressed, and unable to do a day's work.

From that day, I concentrated all my energy and resources to getting better treatment from my doctors and the sleep lab. I demanded and pleaded for earlier appointments. I started to question and take action, adjusting and improving on my face mask, for example. I began to feel energy and hope as I got just a little more sleep. I set myself the goal of finding out how well I could feel with treatment and searching for ways to obtain that treatment.

I am still working on trying to heal and mend the disrupted relationships with friends, family, and associates. I have to accept sadly the realization that some pain and disappointments can never fully be undone nor some relationships recovered.—J.H.

What is required for relief and stability?

Medical and psychological information

When your SAS condition responds to treatment, you may face the need to keep up treatments over the rest of your life. Your response to treatment may be uneven or include dealing with side effects. Recovery may include medical or technological interventions, but these are often only some of several needed components. Compared with the duration of your illness, which may have lasted from 10 to 15 years, the recovery process can proceed at a dizzying pace. In days or weeks of starting effective treatment, normal, refreshing sleep can revitalize the sufferer. A fast-paced recovery and impressive changes in the patient's health may create new problems of readjustment for the patient and those around him or her. To help patients and their families cope with these dramatic developments, support from other patients, the AWAKE organization, a psychologist, or a social worker may be invaluable.

Self-awareness

I must take responsibility for my treatment on a daily basis. I have a broad understanding of the problems related to sleep disorders. I am aware of a range of treatment alternatives and progress being made through research and development on new treatments. I have gained the perspective to interpret my own situation more accurately than before and an intellectual and social basis for emotional stability. This emotional stability helps me ride out temporary setbacks without panicking. Some nights are not restful. I may wake up several times, have a hard time getting back to sleep, or go back to sleep without using the treatment device. I may wake up early but not feel rested enough to get up and do something, yet I may get no benefit from staying in bed. I may oversleep, wake up with a headache, or feel exhausted and down during the day. Even two or three nights of poor sleep can bring back symptoms such as inefficiency, paranoia, and automatic behavior. Recently I spent several hours trying to fix a broken copier, putting the same work into the copier and then opening the copier to clear up the jams. I could have done the copying some other place and finished the task in an hour or two. But I was too tired to realize what was happening.

To treat each of these problems in perspective, I remind myself that they are signs of poor sleep. Therefore, probably something can be done to isolate and correct the cause. Perhaps more importantly, I know that this disaster has a remedy, so I can focus on corrective action and not waste energy on feelings of panic and anxiety. I know that I need review of my sleep hygiene and to check that the treatment device is correctly adjusted and operating properly. I check if I have been taking medications that could affect my sleep. If I cannot solve the problem in a couple of days of trial and error, I may discuss it with my doctor.

Social support

I have created an informed, supportive network of colleagues and friends including professionals and sleep apnea patients. This growing network of others with common concerns gives me much personal and emotional satisfaction. During the initial periods of treatment, I worked with a psychologist. However, perhaps the most helpful experience was my first talk with a fellow patient. Speaking with him was incredibly liberating, showing me that many problems I experienced coping with daily life were like his problems. By talking with other patients with sleep disorders, I learned that they also found it hard to get to morning appointments on time. I realized that I had a handicap rather than a moral defect. Finally I could stop criticizing myself for not meeting social and personal standards of behavior. I began to stand up to my friends and relatives who moralized and gave me advice that I could not follow. Meeting other patients helped me to focus on the real problem: getting relief from the disease. This focus reinforced my determination to put all my energy into getting a proper night's sleep. I was ready to sleep like a bat, hanging from my heels, if that would have helped. My determination and persistence have paid off with the help of my doctors, technicians, home care company, and sleep center.

You can be helped by others and help others.

Other patients may have solved a problem that prevents getting the maximum benefit from the therapy, or they may have valuable experiences in dealing with health maintenance organizations (HMO) or insurance companies. We need each other. That's why we recommend joining (or founding) a mutual help group.

The health-care system can care for you better if you know what you need and how to get it. Your disease is neither a punishment nor the result of weak moral fiber or laziness. Doctors and other professionals in the health-care system are dedicated but fallible men and women—if you are informed and cooperate with them, you improve your chances for recovery. The adversary is ignorance, carelessness, and lack of a rational insurance system. The institutions and individuals with whom you may have to struggle in seeking proper diagnosis and effective treatment are also your allies and partners who want you to recover and succeed. Your efforts and determination will make the difference in your recovery.

If you have untreated severe sleep apnea, you may be barely capable of understanding much of the material in this book. You may be unwilling to admit to the seriousness of the disease and its crippling impact. You may need to be led and supported through the initial phases of recognition, evaluation, and treatment. However, a few days or weeks after your treatment begins and your intellectual capabilities return, you may become a full and active partner in your own treatment. At some points you may be both helpless from the symptoms of prolonged sleep deprivation and terrified that the treatment may not work, and therefore need professional intervention and support. At other times you can become an effective leader and guide to others.

The need for ritual

Successful treatment can lead to major, positive changes in all areas of life. Change may come easily or may involve effort and painful and difficult moments as you readjust your relationships with others and mourn for the losses caused by the disabilities related to sleep disorders. Modern society lacks rituals to mark our reentry into health, so we must rediscover traditional rites or find new ways to celebrate passages and transitions.

Some cultures have maintained a more complex and supportive system of belief which is compatible with scientific medicine. For instance, Navaho Native Americans gather together the friends, relatives, and community of a sick person and use rituals, communal action, and belief in an effort which will restore the community as well as the patient. They believe that disease is an expression of being out of harmony with the natural order, and therefore involve the community as well as the patient in the effort to restore health and well-being to all.

Another model is seen in a short, monthly service in a synagogue attended by physicians and other care givers as well as patients. A small booklet created by service-goers at Temple Israel in Boston, located in the midst of several medical institutions, is titled *Tefillat Refuat Hanefesh, The Service for the Healing of the Soul*. The service begins with remembering the hardships of illness on the person and their loved ones. The middle section seeks help to manage the burdens of illness, and the final section seeks to transcend illness and achieve peace.

In our money-oriented, high-technology society, we look for material answers to every problem. But experiences of sickness and health, frustration and hope, remind us of the simple human truths expressed in religious systems. We need health, an honorable source of income, and a network of loving relationships. We need to recognize that while we attempt to direct and control our lives, we also need to realize that some things are beyond our control or understanding. Medical technology is vital to recover from sleep apnea, but that it is only part of the story of recovery.

Support of loved ones

The spouse, child, friend, or colleague of an SAS patient can play an important role in recovery through understanding, patience, and support. Sleep disorders are insidious and poorly understood. Understanding the medical, technical, and psychological issues confronting the sleep apnea syndrome patient can enable loved ones to contribute to the patient's recovery.

Many symptoms and effects of a sleep disorder can make a patient hard to live with and seem lazy, unreliable, and uninterested in work or other people. However, SAS patients are not lazy, immoral, shiftless, and uncaring. Rather, they are always exhausted, which affects their mental abilities and emotions.

SAS is a handicap that can be overcome with appropriate treatment. Successful treatment for sleep apnea removes nearly all of the symptoms and effects, so loved ones can look forward to the sufferer returning to normal as treatment works. The most important thing is for the person suffering from sleep apnea to get professional advice, diagnosis, and treatment.

Loved ones can support and encourage the patient to seek and follow medical advice. This challenge to the loved ones' patience and ingenuity creates stresses in an already difficult relationship. Many victims of SAS become encased in a shell that is hard to penetrate. This shell is due to the result of pro-longed sleep loss, with a consequent loss of judgment and perspective and attendant fatigue, apathy, discouragement, and depression. In addition, many people have difficulty recognizing the need for help and reaching out for assistance.

Close friends and family members can help the SAS patient adapt to a renewed sense of well-being and energy and a more positive outlook. A change for the better can itself become a temporary problem because the patient may be full of regrets and feel depressed as he or she realizes how much time has been lost and that other people may have been hurt badly. Both loved ones and the patient need to work through these and other issues—including the loved ones' feelings—to build a new relationship meaningful to both people. Professional advice will ease adjustments to changing relationships.

The patient's spouse, family, or friends may find it helpful to attend support group meetings with the patient—to find others with similar experiences and problems who can share with and help each other.

Actors in your new life

Many actors appear in the treatment and rehabilitation process. Knowing these roles will enable you to be a more effective actor and director in the play that determines the rest of your life.

- Physicians diagnose, prescribe medications and treatment, and coordinate paraprofessionals and medical specialists.
- Sleep disorders centers and laboratories provide information, diagnosis, and treatment trials.
- Home care delivery companies and personnel provide equipment, training in its use, and advice and support during the adjustment process.
- Psychologists and other mental-health professionals provide a path of intervention, understanding, realignment of personal and social relations, and support.
- Family, friends, employers, and associates need to adapt to the patient's adjustments in every area of social life.
- Patient or consumer support groups (such as AWAKE) provide information, models based on experience, and valuable perspectives.
- Pastors, rabbis, ministers, priests, imams, healers are people who may be able to respond to the patient's extraordinary feelings and changes in experience, feeling, and status related to the recovery process.
- You, the patient, might need to assess and deal with what can be changed and what might not be capable of recovery, and undertake changes in attitude, habits, and expectations consistent with your new reality.

Confronting adversity

We must each try to understand and control our fate. Acceptance of reality, including our limitations, is the beginning of growth and meaningful adaptation. Psychology recognizes the importance to growth and satisfaction in life of making a sustained, focused effort to overcome obstacles. This effort may be the key to your creating a new, more satisfying life. No less important is the realization that not everything is within our power and control. The nature and limitations of our health-care system requires you to take charge of healing yourself. You can prevail and experience the miracle of adequate rest, health, and recovery of your capacities. Don't let your nightly struggle rob you of another day of your life. If, like me, you have this SAS disease, condition, or syndrome—so often invisible and unrecognized except by the damage it causes—there is hope.

Appendix A

Directory

Organizations

American Sleep Apnea Association, 1424 K Street NW, Suite 302, Washington DC 20005; Tel: 202/293-3650, Fax: 202/293-3656.
<www.sleepapnea.org> *Research, training, education, and advocacy for health professionals and patients with SAS. Newsletter for patients. The A. W. A. K. E. network is the patient education and support program of the ASAA.*

American Sleep Disorders Association, 1610-14th Street NW #300, Rochester, MN 55901. Tel: 507/287-6006 Fax: 507/287-6008 <www.asda.org> *Standards and accreditation, education, advocacy, and information for medical institutions and professionals involved in clinical care of patients with sleep disorders. Publications of the ASDA should be obtained through the National Sleep Foundation.*

A.P.N.E.A. NET (The Apnea Patient's News, Education & Awareness Network) Dave Hargett <www.apneanet.org> <webmaster@apneanet.org> *Providing news and education to sleep apnea patients and their family members, and increasing public awareness of sleep apnea through patient activism.*

Associated Partnership of Sleep Societies, contact through the American Sleep Disorders Association. *An umbrella organization for professional organizations involved in sleep disorders: researchers, clinicians, and sleep polysomnographers.*

Australasian Sleep Society, John Robert Wheatley, MD., Ph.D., Secretary; Department of Respiratory Medicine, Westmead Hospital, 2145 Westmead, NSW, Australia; Tel: 61-2-633-6797; FAX: 61-2-893-9060. *An organization engaged in sleep research, treatment, and education at the professional level.*

A. W. A. K. E. Network: *Groups providing information, mutual help and support, and advocacy for persons with SAS and other sleep-related breathing disorders, and for their families.* For information, contact American Sleep Apnea Association.

British Snoring and Sleep Apnoea Association, Allen D. Davey, Director, 0737-557-997, The Steps, How Lane, Chipstead, Surrey CR5 3LT, England. *Education, support, newsletter for patients and professionals.*

Canadian Sleep Society (CSS), Rachel L. Morehouse, MD., ACP, FRCP, Secretary, Sleep Disorders Lab, Camp Hill Medical Centre, Room 4008, Abbie Lane Building, 1763 Robie St., Halifax, Nova Scotia B3H 3G2, Canada; FAX: 902/492-4779. *An organization engaged in sleep research, treatment, and education at the professional level.*

European Sleep Research Society (ESRS), Alain Muzet, M.D., contact person, LPPE_CNRS, 21 rue Becquerel, 67087 Strasbourg Cedex, France; FAX: 33-88-10-62-45. *An organization engaged in sleep research, treatment, and education at the professional level.*

Gazette International Networking Institute, Joan L. Headley, Executive Director, 314/534-0475, 5100 Oakland Avenue #206, St. Louis Missouri 63110 USA. *(G.I.N.I. is a network of people providing answers to questions about disability and it publishes journals: topics include rehabilitation and independent living, polio, and muscular dystrophy. See I.V.U.N.)*

International Ventilator Users Network (I.V.U.N.), Joan L. Headley, Executive Director, 314/534-0475, 5100 Oakland Avenue, #206, Saint Louis, Missouri 63110 USA. *An organization that links ventilator users (persons with various breathing disorders) with each other and with health care professionals interested in home mechanical ventilation. Publishes information on nasal masks and other topics that may be helpful to persons with SAS using CPAP. Copies of* the *Directory of Sources for Ventilation Face Masks are $2.50 each but will be sent without charge to anyone in financial difficulty.*

Japanese Society of Sleep Research (JSSR), Mitsukuni Murasaki (Secretary), Department of Neuro-psychiatry, Kitasato University, Higashi Hospital, 863-1 Asamizo-dai 2-1-1, 228 Sagamihara-city, Kanaagawa-Prefecture, Japan; Tel: 81-427-48-9119 *An organization engaged in sleep research, treatment, and education at the professional level.*

Latin American Sleep Society (LASS), Patricio D. Peirano, Contact person, Neurophysiology Unit, Inta-Universidad de Chile, Casilla 138-11, Santiago Chile; FAX: 56-2-221-40-30 *An organization engaged in sleep research, treatment, and education at the professional level.*

MedicAlert Foundation International, Turlock, CA 95381-1009, 800-ID-ALERT. *System to provide emergency medical information by telephone about subscribers who carry or wear an identification bracelet or necklace.*

Narcolepsy Network, POB 4260, Cincinnati OH 45242, Tel: 513/891-3522, Fax: 513/991-9936 <www.websciences.org/narnet> <narnet@aol.com> *National, non-profit organization whose members are people who have narcolepsy (or related sleep disorders), their families and friends, and professionals involved in treatment, research, and public education regarding narcolepsy.*

National Center on Sleep Disorders Research (NCSDR), 2 Rock Ledge Center, Suite 10038, Bethesda, MD 20892; Tel: 301/435-0199 Fax: 301/480-3451. <www.nhlbi.nih.gov/nhlbi/sleep/sleep.htm> Director, Dr. James Kiley. *Coordination, research, training, education, and technology transfer in sleep disorders and sleep.*

National Commission on Sleep Disorders Research, Stanford University Sleep Disorders Center, 701 Welch Rd., Suite 2226, Palo Alto, CA 94304; 415/725-6484; FAX 415/725-7341. *Reported to NIH, Congress, and the President on needs* and priorities in sleep disorders research.

Restless Legs Syndrome Foundation, 4410 19th Street NW - Suite 201, Rochester MN 55901-6624 <www.rls.org> <rlsf@millcomm.com> *Provides information about RLS; helps develop support groups; supports research to find better treatments and, eventually, a definitive cure; educates physicians and patients about RLS; and publishes a quarterly newsletter known as* NightWalkers.

Wake Up America! 701 Welch Rd., Suite 2226, Palo Alto, CA 94304; Tel: 415/723-8131 Fax: 415/725-7341 Contact: Mike Davis; William C. Dement, M.D., Ph.D., Chairman. *Awareness and action towards needs and priorities in sleep disorders.*

National Sleep Foundation (NSF), 729 15th Street NW, 4th Floor, Washington, DC 20005. <www.sleepfoundation.org> *Research, information, and education related to sleep disorders for the public and media.*

NORD—National Organization for Rare Disorders, POB 8923, New Fairfield, CT 06812, 203/746-6518. *Information, advocacy, and networking for many disorders which are little-known or which affect a small number of persons.*

Sleep/Wake Disorders Canada and the Canadian Association for Narcolepsy, Station S, Toronto ON M5M4L7 Canada, 1-800-387-9253; 416/398-1627. *A national voluntary organization dedicated to helping people suffering from sleep/wake disorders.*

Sleep Apnea Help & Support Group, POBox 351, Pietermartizburg, 3200 South Africa; Tel: 0331-421-913, FAX: 0331-452-162; Attention: Annelte Van Rensburg. *Motto: "To understand, to share, to motivate, to spread knowledge, while living a quality life."*

Sleep Disorders Australia (SDA), Mr. Laurie Cree, President, 102 Pacific Highway, POB 303, Roseville NSW 2069, Australia; Tel: 61-2-9415-6300, FAX: 61-2-9416-9727. *This active patient support group publishes a newsletter and distributes* Phantom of the Night *in Australia, New Zealand, and South East Asian markets.*

Sleep Apnoea Trust, Dieter Shaw, Chairman, Warwick Lodge, Piddington Lane, Piddington, High Wycombe, Bucks HP14 3BD, England; Tel: (44) +01494-881-369, FAX: 011-44-0895-449-849. <www.net.link.co.uk/users/jja/sat> <satrust@aol.com> *A charitable trust involved in education and support for the patient and creating public awareness; collaborates with clinics, hospitals, and manufacturers throughout Great Britain; publishes a newsletter and a video.*

Sleep Disorders Dental Society, 11676 Perry Highway, Building 1, Suite 1204, Wexford PA 15090

Stanford University Sleep Apnea Awareness Project, Stanford University Sleep Research Center, 701 Welch Road, Suite 2226, Palo Alto, CA 94304; 415/725-8920; FAX: 415/725-7341; *Training and support in sleep disorders medicine, especially sleep apnea syndrome, for primary care physicians and other health care professionals in their practices. A variety of training is available, including a three-hour CME course; grand rounds presentations at participating hospitals; individual tutuorials; and technical training in the use of ambulatory monitoring equipment. Dr. Riccardo Stoohs, director of the Stanford Human Sleep Research Lab, is available to assist all health care professionals as part of the program of training and support.*

Manufacturers

Manufacturers of Monitoring and Diagnostic Equipment

Aequitron Medical Inc., Customer & Technical Support, 14800 28th Ave. North, Minneapolis, MN 55447; Tel: 800/497-4979 FAX: 612/557-8200

Astromed-Grass Instrument Company, Mr. Ed Johnson, Applications Engineer, 600 E. Greenwich Ave., West Warwick, RI 02893; 800/225-5167.

Nellcor Puritan Bennett has been acquired by Mallinkrodt. Global Sleep Solutions Group, 2800 Northwest Boulevard, Minneapolis MN 55441-2625; Tel: 612/694-3500; 800/497-4979, customer service: 800/497-4968, Fax: 612/694-3547 <www.mallinckrodt.com> <www.nellcorpb.com> Diagnostic devices include apnea screening devices, pulse oximeters. Software for analysis of diagnostic and treatment studies.

Nicolet Instrument Corporation, David L. Stephenson, Director of Marketing, Biomedical Division, 5225 Verona Rd., Madison, Wisconsin 53711-4495; 608/271-3333, Fax 608/273-5067

Nihon Kohden America, Ms. Adrian DeGuire, Product Manager, 2601 Campus Drive, Irvine CA 92715; 800/325-0283

Oxford Medical, Inc., Ms. Sandy Cleenney, Sales Manager, Neurophysiology, 11526 53rd North St., Clearwater FLA 813/573-4500

SensorMedics Corporation, 22705 Savi Ranch Parkway, Yorba Linda CA 92687, Tel: 714-283-1830, 800/520-4368, FAX 714/283-8493 <www.sensormedics.com>

Synectics Medical, 1425 Greenway Drive, Irving TX 75038, 1-800/227-3191; FAX 214/518-0080

TeleDiagnostic Systems, Mr. Larry Reis, 2053 Sutter St., San Francisco CA 94115, 1-800/227-3224

Telefactor Corp., Mr. Alfredo Bustamente, Union Hill Building, DeHaven St. W Consoohocken PA 19428, 215/825-4555

Vitalog Monitoring, Inc., Dr. Laughton Miles, 643 Bair Island Road Suite 212, Redwood City CA 94063; 413/366-8676; FAX: 415/368-5779

Manufacturers of treatment devices, equipment, and supplies

AirSep Corporation, 401 Creekside Drive, Buffalo NY 14228-2085; Tel: 716/874-0202, 800/874-0202; Fax: 716/691-4141 <www.airsep.com> Treatment device: Remedy® CPAP; masks and accessories; Ultimate™ mask can use a gel interface.

Sunrise Medical/DeVilbiss, Respiratory Products Division, Mr. Mark D'Angelo, Director, Sleep Business Unit, P.O.Box. 635, Somerset PA 15501-0635; customer service: 800/333-4000; FAX 800/847-3291. <www.sunrisemedical.com/apnea.html> <info@dhc-sunmed.com> Horizon™ brand, devices include CPAP, BiLevel, AutoAdjust, and a treatment monitor/recorder.

Healthdyne Technologies has been acquired by Respironics, Inc. The former Healthdyne facility is at 1255 Kennestone Circle, Marietta, GA 30066; for customer service, call 800/333-4000 or contact Respironics, Inc.

LifeCare International has been acquired by Respironics, Inc. For customer satisfaction, call 800/669-9234 or contact Respironics, Inc.

Medical Industries America, Inc., 2879 R Ave., Adel IA 50003-9719; 800/759-3038 Fax 515/913-4172 Treatment device: CPAP

Nellcor Puritan Bennett has been acquired by Mallinkrodt. Global Sleep Solutions Group, 2800 Northwest Boulevard, Minneapolis MN 55441-2625; Tel: 612/694-3500; 800/497-4979, customer service: 800/497-4968, Fax: 612/694-3547 <www.mallinckrodt.com> <www.nellcorpb.com> Treatment devices include: CPAP, Bilevel, auto-CPAP (not in USA), masks and accessories, oral appliance; diagnostic devices include apnea screening devices, pulse oximiters. Software for analysis of diagnostic and treatment studies.

Nidek Medical Products, Inc., 3949 Valley East Industrial Drive, Birmingham AL 35217; Tel: 205/856-7200, 800/822-9255; Fax: 205/856-0533. <www.nidekmedical.com> Treatment devices: Silenzio® CPAP, Silenzio® Plus CPAP/Bilevel

ResMed, Inc., Dr. Peter Farrell, President/CEO; 10121 Carroll Canyon Rd., San Diego CA 92131-1109; Customer Support: Tel: 1-800/424-0737, FAX: 619/880-1618. <www.resmed.com> Treatment devices: Sullivan® brand of CPAP (3), Sullivan Bilevel (2); Auto-Set® system models combine diagnosis, titration, and treatment; masks and accessories including heated humidifiers.

Respironics, Inc., 1501 Ardmore Boulevard, Pittsburgh, PA 15221; Customer service, Tel: 800/345-6443, FAX: 800/886-0245. <http://www.respironics.com> Treatment devices: Virtuoso, Aria, Solo brands; CPAP, BiPap™ (bilevel); Virtuoso® LX smart CPAP; masks and accessories; diagnostic and monitoring devices.

Sources of custom and special masks, headgear, and accessories

John Bach, M.D., University of Medicine & Dentistry, University Hospital, Dept. of Rehabilitation B-239, 150 Bergen Street, Newark NJ 07103-2425

Barry Make, M.D., Director, Pulmonary Rehabilitation, National Center for Immunology and Respiratory Medicine, 1400 Jackson Street, Denver CO 80206; 303/398-1783

Hans Rudolph, Inc., 5 Central, Kansas City MO 64114; Tel: 816/363-5522, 800/456-6695; Fax: 816/822-1414; Masks and accessories including full-face masks (for custom research and clinical applications), CPAP nasal masks, headgear, hydro-gel seals for nasal masks.

Hugh Newton-John, M.D., Yarra Bend Road, Fairfield Victoria 3078, Australia

Peter Peschel, Ochtumstrasse 30, Postfach 12 24 2806 Oyten, West Germany

REMAFA Tech, Pilggvagen 34, 126-36 Hagersten, Sweden

SEFAM, Rue Du Bois de la Champelle, 54500 Vandoeuvere-Les-Nancy, France (Distributed by Lifecare)

SleepNet Corporation, Tom Moulton, President, Lockheed Air Center, 1050 Perimeter Road, Manchester, NH 03103; Tel: 603/624-1911; 800/742-3646 Fax: 603/641-9440 <http://www.dpap.com> Treatment accessory: masks.

LifeCare International, has been acquired by Respironics, Inc. For customer satisfaction, call 800/669-9234 or contact Respironics, Inc.

Susan Sortor, RRT, Dallas Rehabilitation Institute, 9713 Harry Hines Blvd., Dallas Texas 75220

Tiara Medical Systems, Inc., 14414 Detroit Ave., Suite 205, Lakewood OH 44107; Tel: 216/521-1220, 800/582-7458, Fax: 216/521-1399

Home care companies

Apria Healthcare, 3560 Hyland Avenue, Costa Mesa, CA 92626; 1-800/APRIA-88

Ambulatory Services of America, 5834 C Peachtree Corners East, Norcross GA 30092, 1-800/950-1580

Amcare Medical Services, Inc., 459 Watertown Street, Newton MA, 02160, 800/669-1970

American Home Patient Centers, 105 Reynolds Drive, Franklin, Tenn.

Hitech Homecare, 5980 East Unity Dr., Norcross GA 30071; Tel: 404-449-6785, 800-449-6785; FAX: 404-449-0648

Kimberley Quality Care, Charlotte Gann, HME Satellite Manager, 600 Century Plaza Drive #165, Houston TX 77073; 713/821-7475

Lincare, Inc., Brian Jennings, General Manager, Sales; 888 Executive Center Drive West, Suite 300, St. Petersburg, FL 33702; Sales Information, 1-800/284-2006 Ext. 207; 813/576-4404.

Med-Care, Inc., 100 Prince St., Kingston NY 12401; Tel: 914/331-2400; FAX: 914/331-2492

Nahatan Medical Services, 129 Lenox St., Norwood MA 02062; Tel 617/769-0404, 800/649-2422; FAX: 617/769-6926

NMC Homecare, a division of National Medical Care, Inc., Jonathan D. Fickett, Business Manager, Respiratory Therapy, 1601 Trapelo Road, Waltham, MA 02154; 617/466-9850, Extension 427; 800/662-1237, Extension 427.

Primedica, Steve Sensabaugh, Director of Materials Management, 1841 West Oak Parkway, West Oak Center, Marietta GA 30062, 800/647-3729

Protocare, Karen Mercer, Clinical Director; 950 Winter St., Waltham MA 02154; 617/890-5560

Appendix B

Treating persons with SAS

Confirm with your physician that the information in this Appendix applies correctly to your condition before use. NTP grants permission for the owner of this book to copy this Appendix for his/her personal use including to add it to your medical records and show it to your physician and admitting personnel before admission to hospital.

Medical Information

Airway management may be difficult—avoid sedatives, narcotics, and tranquilizers.
I have obstructive sleep apnea syndrome.

Name:_____

Address:_____

My physician for treatment of apnea is:_____(Tel.)_____

I am currently using nasal CPAP at _____ cm. H_2O.

I use bilevel airway management in _____mode with ipap =_____, epap =_____ cm. H_2O.

© 1995 New Technology Publishing, Inc.

To all medical personnel—airway maintenance

Sleep apnea is caused by a failure of the muscles controlling the upper airway thus the airway collapses and blocks the flow of breath although the muscles of the diaphragm and chest try to breathe. This blockage may be caused by sleep, medications, or alterations in consciousness. While hospitalized or under treatment for other conditions, I should not receive sleeping pills, hypnotics, sedatives or tranquilizers, narcotics, or medications known to affect neuromuscular transmission without due consideration for maintenance of my airway.

Continuing CPAP during hospitalization

Should I be receiving home respiratory support such as nasal CPAP, it should be continued during my hospitalization under the direction of my physician.

Cautions Before Surgical, Medical, Dental or Radiological Procedures

If you are admitted to a hospital or are undergoing any dental, surgical, or medical procedure that may involve the use of a painkiller, anesthesia, or relaxing medication, you should take precautions. Inform each of your doctors and dentists and make sure that they understand the risks involved in procedures on patients with sleep apnea. You may want to copy this information and make it part of your medical records.

Snoring as a risk factor

The most risky situation is one without suspicion of sleep-related breathing abnormality. If you snore loudly, but don't know if you have sleep apnea, bring it to the attention of your surgeon and anesthesiologist before surgery.

Procedures with sedation

Many procedures performed on both inpatients and outpatients utilize sedation. These include but are not limited to endoscopy, special radiologic procedures (CT, MRI), routine surgery, and dental procedures. Numerous medications used in such circumstances may cause the upper airway to collapse leading to upper airway obstruction. Such obstruction could prove fatal. You must inform physicians, technicians, nurses, or other personnel of this risk so that they can take necessary precautions. An important indication to you that drugs may be utilized or needed in any procedure is the placement of an intravenous line. The placement of such a line should remind you to inform the personnel that your airway may be hard to manage.

Dental procedures

Dental procedures do not commonly require intravenous medications but oral sedatives and/or the use of nitrous oxide (laughing gas) should also be undertaken with appropriate precautions.

Risks in surgery

The risk of surgery to patients with sleep apnea is much greater than in normal individuals. This warning is true regardless of the purpose or type of surgery. The risk is that the patient under surgery will not be able to breathe as the result of loss of control over the throat muscles, which may relax and block the air passage.

It is general practice to anesthetize the patient, usually with intravenous anesthesia, before an endotracheal tube (a breathing tube that fits into the throat and trachea) is placed into the windpipe for the delivery of general anesthesia and to maintain breathing during the operation. In the apnea patient, disastrous results can ensue before the anesthesiologist has placed the breathing tube into the airway. The patient becomes unconscious, the muscles of the throat relax, and the extremely relaxed tissues of the upper airway collapse, making it difficult if not impossible to put the endotracheal tube into the windpipe. The patient may be unable to breathe; sometimes the only way out of this life-threatening situation is to perform an emergency tracheostomy.

Postoperative considerations

After surgery, the immediate postoperative period is also a risky time for obstruction since patients usually require pain medication. Vigilant monitoring should include the use of an apnea monitor and oximeter. Regional anesthesia (preferably without narcotics) should be used when possible for pain control. Nasal CPAP or other respiratory support is often needed postoperatively. Surgery on the upper airway or neck may compound the risks because of the swelling of the tissues that accompany the procedure.

Emergency information

MedicAlert

MedicAlert emblems carry identification which can enable medical personnel to quickly obtain information about you in an emergency. To register, contact the MedicAlert Foundation International, Turlock, CA 95381-1009, 800-ID-ALERT. We suggest the following information be entered:

- Emblem Information—**sleep apnea syndrome**

Additional emergency medical information—**airway management may be difficult—avoid sedatives, narcotics, tranquilizers**

Information Card

Verify with your physician that this information is valid for you before use. NTP grants permission for the owner of this book to copy this Appendix for his/her personal use. Complete and sign, then cut out both pieces, place them back-to-back and align, then secure with clear tape. To seal, use wide, clear package sealing tape to enclose front and back, or any commercially available lamination method. Fold to fit wallet or purse.

✂

Emergency Medical Information

Airway management may be difficult—avoid sedatives, narcotics, and tranquilizers.

I have **obstructive sleep apnea**

I am at risk of a blockage or cessation of breathing that could lead to death if:
- I lose consciousness for any reason.
- I take a drug that causes drowsiness or sedation or muscle relaxation.
- I undergo a dental, surgical, or diagnostic procedure in which anesthesia is used.
-

Because of my condition it may be extremely difficult to perform endotracheal intubation.

Should I require airway support or management take all due precautions and attempt to intubate without sedation, general anesthesia, or muscle relaxants if possible.

I carry this card to authorize emergency aid or treatment should I be unable to supply this information myself.

_____(Signed)

© 1995 New Technology Publishing, Inc.

Emergency Medical Information

Airway management may be difficult—avoid sedatives, narcotics, and tranquilizers.

I have **obstructive sleep apnea syndrome.**

Name:_____

Address:_____

My physician for treatment of apnea is:_____(Tel.)_____
My personal physician is:_____(Tel.)_____
Family member to contact_____(Tel.)_____
I am currently using nasal CPAP at _____ cm. H_2O.
I use bi-level airway management in _____ mode with ipap =_____, epap =_____ cm. H_2O.

© 1995 New Technology Publishing, Inc.

Appendix C

Sleep log form

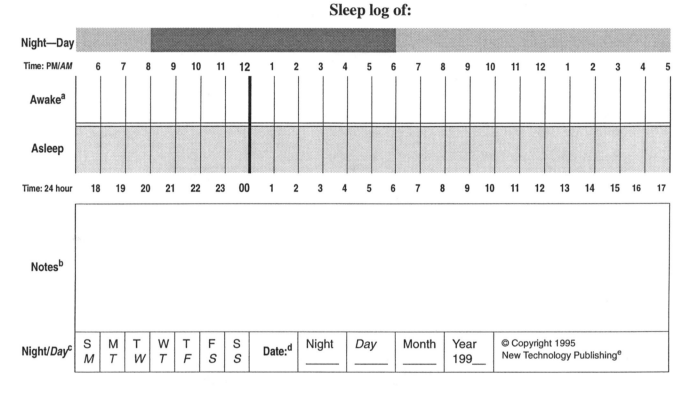

Sleep log of:

a. Draw a horizontal line that is in the awake zone for the time when you are awake, and in the asleep zone when you take a nap or are sleeping. If you take a nap during the day, the line would dip down during the nap. If you wake up during the night, the line should rise up into the awake zone.

b. Record how you felt during the day: alert, drowsy, naps taken. How was your functioning and level of performance? Any symptoms of sleepiness? How did you sleep? Any awakenings? What medications? Exercise? Any other issues that might affect your sleep or be affected by it. You can make additional comments and observations in a separate diary or additional pages.

c. Circle the pair of letters that represent the combination of the name of the day when you go to sleep and the day you arise. For example, you go to sleep on Sunday night and wake up on Monday morning, so you would mark the first pair.

d. Enter the date of the night you go to sleep and the day you awake.

e. The purchaser or owner of this book may make copies of this sleep log form for his/her personal use, or additional copies can be obtained from New Technology Publishing.

Sleep log of:

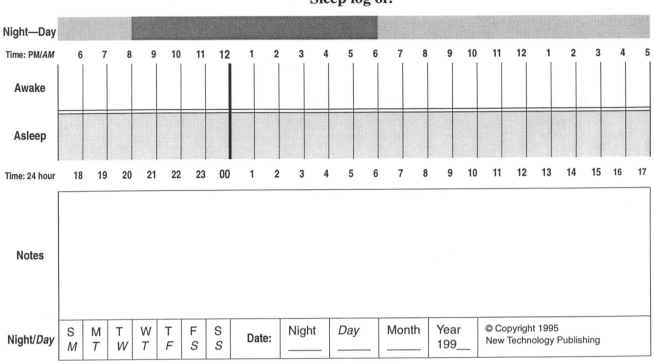

Sleep log of:

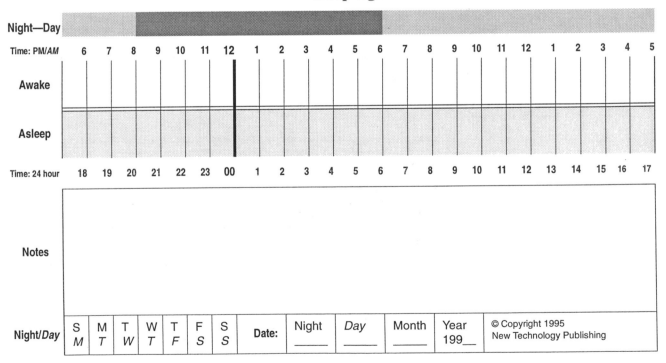

Sleep log of:

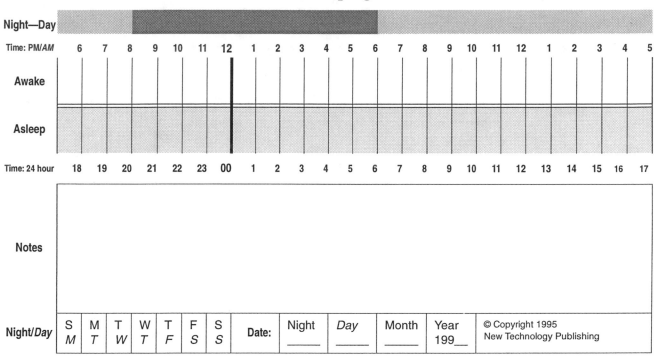

Night—Day

| Time: PM/*AM* | 6 | 7 | 8 | 9 | 10 | 11 | 12 | 1 | 2 | 3 | 4 | 5 | 6 | 7 | 8 | 9 | 10 | 11 | 12 | 1 | 2 | 3 | 4 | 5 |

Awake

Asleep

| Time: 24 hour | 18 | 19 | 20 | 21 | 22 | 23 | 00 | 1 | 2 | 3 | 4 | 5 | 6 | 7 | 8 | 9 | 10 | 11 | 12 | 13 | 14 | 15 | 16 | 17 |

Notes

| Night/*Day* | S M | M T | T W | W T | T F | F S | S S | Date: | Night ____ | *Day* ____ | Month ____ | Year 199__ | © Copyright 1995 New Technology Publishing |

Sleep log of:

Night—Day

| Time: PM/*AM* | 6 | 7 | 8 | 9 | 10 | 11 | 12 | 1 | 2 | 3 | 4 | 5 | 6 | 7 | 8 | 9 | 10 | 11 | 12 | 1 | 2 | 3 | 4 | 5 |

Awake

Asleep

| Time: 24 hour | 18 | 19 | 20 | 21 | 22 | 23 | 00 | 1 | 2 | 3 | 4 | 5 | 6 | 7 | 8 | 9 | 10 | 11 | 12 | 13 | 14 | 15 | 16 | 17 |

Notes

| Night/*Day* | S M | M T | T W | W T | T F | F S | S S | Date: | Night ____ | *Day* ____ | Month ____ | Year 199__ | © Copyright 1995 New Technology Publishing |

Sleep log of:

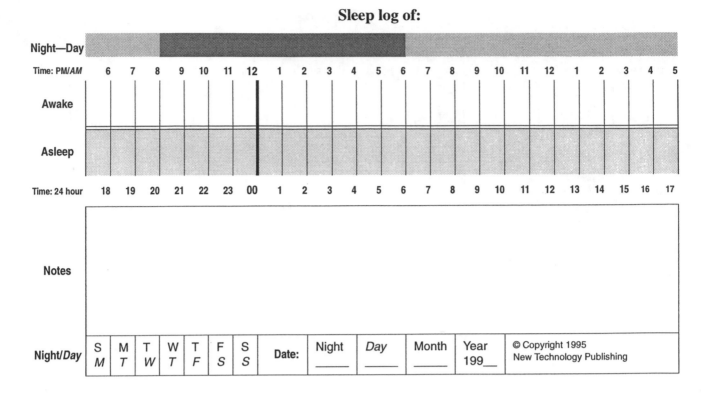

| S M | M T | T W | W T | T F | F S | S S | Date: | Night ___ | *Day* ___ | Month ___ | Year 199__ | © Copyright 1995 New Technology Publishing |

Sleep log of:

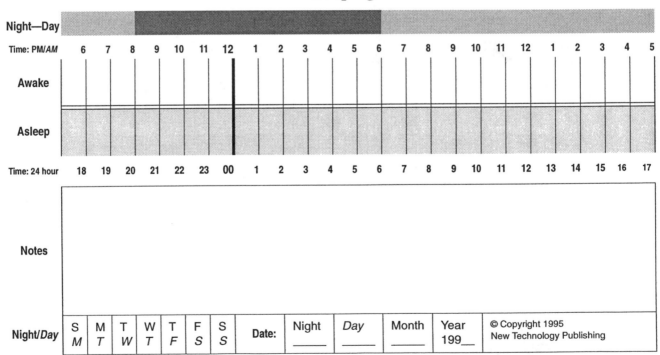

| S M | M T | T W | W T | T F | F S | S S | Date: | Night ___ | *Day* ___ | Month ___ | Year 199__ | © Copyright 1995 New Technology Publishing |

Appendix D

Equipment and accessories

Table D.1   CPAP treatment devices and accessories[a]

	Ramp feature	Filter	Size & weight	Electrical	Accessories & Special Features
AirSep Remedy® CPAP	Specifications not available at press time				Ultimate® Nasal Mask, optional gel seal
Healthdyne® Technologies: Tranquility Quest™ CPAP	0-30 (increments of 5 minutes)	Reusable, washable foam; optional high grade disposable	4.5 inches H x 9.5L x 7.75 W (10.8 cm x 23.6 x 18.9); 4.5 lbs(2.1 kg)	Automatic switching for 100-240 VAC, 50/60 Hz. Optional 12 VDC to AC inverter.	Soft Series™ and standard masks (7 sizes); nasal seal as alternative to mask; hose length options of 6 or 10 feet; oxygen administration kit; humidifier; DC power cord Two-year warranty, optional third year. **This unit is still available. Healthdyne has been acquired by Respironics, Inc.**
Medical Industries America, Inc. Sleepap	Linear ramp, adjustable from 6-54 minutes in 6-minute intervals	Reusable foam	8 inches H x 8W x 12 D; 6.1 pounds; 20 cm x 20 x 30; 2.29 kg	120 VAC, 60 Hz; or 220 VAC, 50 Hz	Three types of masks and headgear; ADAM circuit; manometer; case.
Nellcor Puritan Bennett: GoodKnight™ 318 (CPAP)	0,5,10 or 20 minute delay before ramping up to prescribed pressure	Reusable high-efficiency filter	4 inches H x 9 W x 11D;10 cm. x 22.9 x 27.9; 5.3 lbs./2.4 kg.	100-240 VAC, 50/60 Hz DC to AC inverter available	LED light bar indicates CPAP pressure. Options: compliance meter. Humidifier, carrying case, manometer assembly, oxygen adapter; ADAM circuit nasal pillow system; nasal masks in 3 sizes; Sullivan® nasal bubble masks. Quiet (sound output 38 dBA, 10 cm water pressure at 1 meter), light. Two-year warranty.
Nellcor Puritan Bennett: GoodKnight™ 314 (CPAP)	Clinician-adjustable ramp start pressure with 20 minute delay.	Reusable high-efficiency filter	4 inches H x 9 W x 11D;10 cm. x 22.9 x 27.9; 5.3 lbs./2.4 kg.	115 VAC, 50/60 Hz. DC to AC inverter available	Quiet (sound output 38 dBA, 10 cm water pressure at 1 meter), light. Two-year warranty. Optional compliance meter indicates time spent breathing on unit.

Table D.1 CPAP treatment devices and accessories[a]

	Ramp feature	Filter	Size & weight	Electrical	Accessories & Special Features
ResMed Sullivan® V Nasal CPAP Systems (V, V Plus, V Elite)	Delay selected by patient: 0, 5, 10, 20 minutes (up to maximum set by technician)	Polyester fibre 1 in./ 24 mm thick	4.15 in x 9.5 x 11 in; 10.5 cm H x 24 W x 28 cm. L; 4.5 pounds/ 2 kg	Universal power supply with automatic switching for 110-240 V, 50-400 Hz; 80 VA max; 24 VDC (battery)	**Sullivan® Mirage mask system.** Lightweight, low profile, stable mask and headgear system for comfort, low noise, secure seal. **Sullivan® special application Nose and Mouth mask system,** adding mouth cushion to standard or bubble cushion. Two types of Sullivan® bubble cushion mask & three types of headgear, frames; disposable humidification mask insert; **HumidAire™ heated humidifier;** 24 V and 12/24 VDC converters All three models of this system have delay timer, are microprocessor-controlled, self-testing, and can download compliance data. *Sullivan V Plus* adds pressure indicator. *Sullivan V Elite also* adds SmartStart™ to activate system only while patient is using the mask; can download actual usage data; pressure feedback to compensate for atmospheric pressure/ altitude changes or mask leaks. Convenient for travel, quiet, light. Overall noise level at 1 m at 10 cm output pressure, less than 43dB(A); at 20 cm output pressure, less than 50dB(A). Two-year warranty.
Respironics Solo™ and Solo Plus CPAP systems	20	Reusable filter screens pollen & dust. Ultra-fine filter is optional addition for allergens and small particles.	10.0 inches x 5.55 x 4.25 (25 x 14 x 11 cm); ~5 lb./ 2.27 kg.	115 VAC/230 VAC; 12 VDC	**The Monarch™ Mini Mask** is a nasal interface available for use with any CPAP system. The small, lightweight mask is held against the lower surface of the nose by a headgear incorporating flexible pieces which encircle the ear. The mask does not obstruct vision and allows the patient to use eyeglasses. The **Comfort Seal™ Mask Accessory** conforms to the contours of the nose for comfort and to reduce or eliminate leaks. **Spectrum™ Disposable Full Face Mask** is an alternative to nasal masks in CPAP or bi-level therapy for obstructive sleep apnea, and is intended to overcome the effects of mouth leaks. Pressure adjustment to compensate for elevation. Plus has meter to monitor patient usage.
Respironics®: Aria® LX CPAP System	0-45 minutes, therapist adjusts ramp-up time in 5-minute increments. Patient can use ramp button to re-start ramp at low pressure.	Pollen and ultra-fine (optional); filter area about 8.75 square inches	11.66" x 6.75" x 5.40" (30x17 x 14 cm.) 3.5 lbs. (1.6 kg)	Auto-ranging power supply adapts to 115 VAC, 60 Hz; 230 VAC, 50 Hz; 12 VDC; class II, Type B.	The Aria has a microprocessor-driven LCD screen with separate menus for patient and therapist. Therapist can control pressure, ramp length and starting pressure, can access patient usage information and set option to alert patient if mask is accidentally removed. Patient can access the mask removal indicator. Patient can view but not change pressure settings, compliance meter, and total operation time. System can store two years of usage information. Compensates for variations in elevation and leaks and works at atmospheric pressures of 83-102 kPascals and at elevations of 0-5,500 ft. (0-1.67 km). Sound output less than 54 dB for pressure range of 3-20 cm H_2O. System automatically starts and stops in response to patient putting on mask & breathing. Two-year warranty.

Table D.1 CPAP treatment devices and accessories[a]

	Ramp feature	Filter	Size & weight	Electrical	Accessories & Special Features
Sunrise/DeVilbiss: Horizon™LT and STandard Nasal CPAP Systems	20 minute delay, startup pressure is adjustable	Washable, reusable	LT: 7.7 inches W x 4 H x 10.2 D, 3.6 lbs./ 1.6kg STandard: 9.75 inches W x 9.75H x 7.25 D (25cm x 25 x 18;) 6.7 lbs/3 kg.	100-240 VAC, 50/60 Hz	Headgear: strap and cap versions; Masks include silicone, ultra thin membrane, DeVilbiss Seal-Ring™ for comfort, leak-resistance, gel cushion with flexible frame. Humidifiers (passover and heated). Utilization meter records when unit is at pressure; breathing activated start-up (shuts down when not in use); two-year warranty.Healthcare professionals can use the Surveyor™ monitor to do one-night respiratory-event studies or to track a history of patient usage. LT also can interface with SMART *Track*™ modem to monitor patient usage during intitial treatment. ST has microprocessor blower control, automatic startup/shutdown, interface to clinical remote, upgradeable to AutoAdjust and BiLevel.
Sunrise/DeVilbiss Horizon BiLevel™	0,10,20,30 minute delay	Washable, re-usable, foam	9.75 inches W x 9.75H x 7.25 D (25cm x 25 x 18;) 8 lb./ 3/6 kg.	100-240 VAC, 50/60 Hz	Independent control of inspiratory and expiratory breathing cycles to increase patient comfort and enhance clinical value. Each cycle can be adjusted for patient comfort 365-day history of usage records time while patient is using device. Compatible with surveyor.
Nellcor Puritan Bennett: KnightStar™ 320 I/E and 320B (bi-level respiratory systems)	Patient-adjustable 0-30 minute delay before ramping up to prescribed pressure	Washable	7 inches H x 9 W x 7.5 D;18 cm. x 23 x 19; weighs 8.5 lbs/ 3.7 kg.	120 VAC, 50-60 Hz	Humidifier, carrying case, DC power cord, manometer assembly, oxygen adapter; ADAM circuit nasal pillow system; nasal masks in 3 sizes; Sullivan® nasal bubble masks. Infrared remote control. KnightStar 320 and 320B are bi-level respiratory systems providing adjustable sensitivity to synchronize inhale and exhale flow with patient. The 320B model can be set to force a breath if not initiated by the patient. One-year warranty.
ResMed Sullivan® Nasal Sullivan®VPAP II® System Sullivan® VPAP II ST (timed) Sullivan® Comfort (bi-level pressure)	Delay selected by patient: 0, 5, 10, 20 minutes	Polyester/ foam 1 in./ 24 mm thick	5.7 in x 9.4 x 13.8; 14.5 cm H x 24.0 W x 35.0 L; 9.1 pounds/ 4.1 kg	Universal power supply with automatic switching for 110-240 V, 50-400 Hz; 24 VDC (battery)	**For masks, see ResMed Sullivan V listing.** 24 V and 12/24 VDC converters; factory recommends specifically for this unit the Radio Shack Inverter, US# 22-132A, Canada # 12-20 (confirm before using!) Ultra-quiet operation. SmartStart™ to activate system only while patient is using the mask. Smooth transition between pressure levels for comfort. Visual pressure indicator; one-year warranty. Each of three bi-level systems has different specifications and applications.
Nellcor Puritan Bennett® KnightStar™ 335 Respiratory Support System	Delay settable to 0-30 minutes before ramping up to prescribed pressure.	High-efficiency filter system	19 lbs./8.6 kg	115 VAC/240AC; 50-60Hz	Offers three treatment modes: CPAP, positive airway pressure from +3 to +20 cm; bi-level, I/E PAP; Assist/ Control, like the I/E PAP but with back up rate from 3 to 30 breaths per minute. Control module for clinical monitoring.
Respironics BiPAP® Duet® System	0-45 minutes, therapist adjusts. Patient can use ramp button to re-start ramp at low pressure.	Pollen and ultra-fine (optional); filter area about 8.75 square inches	15.25" x 8.75" x 5.40" (39x22x 14cm.) ~12lbs. (5.45 kg)	115 VAC 230 VAC, 12 VDC with DC interface module	Microprocessor LCD screen. Separate pressures for inhalation and exhalation. Automatic compesation for elevation. Automatic on/off controlled by patient breathing. Mask removal warning sound.
Respironics®: BiPAP® S Airway Management System (bi-level pressure)		Disposable 0.3 micron	9.5 lbs./ 4.32 kg	115 VAC/230AC; 12VDC; 12VDC interface module with battery adapter cable	Different pressures for inspiration and expiration

Table D.1   CPAP treatment devices and accessories[a]

	Ramp feature	Filter	Size & weight	Electrical	Accessories & Special Features
ResMed Sullivan® AutoSet® Systems—Clinical, Portable II & Home Models	These three models—Clinical, Portable II, and *AutoSet T* for home use—are intelligent CPAP devices which vary the treatment pressure, attempting to minimize pressure while responding to changing patient needs. The design is intended to provide the lowest effective treatment pressure, which may vary from breath to breath over one night, from night to night, or over a period of months. They are claimed to be comparable to standard professional laboratory CPAP titrations in eliminating apneas, overcoming flow limitations or snoring, and arousals related to respiratory events. {{COLSPAN}} The *AutoSet* systems are programmed to use information about recent breaths, while responding pre-emptively with increased pressure to prevent or overcome an apnea, and to snoring or flow limitation by increasing pressure to avoid a full apnea. The system will respond and attempt to eliminate snoring and silent inspiratory flow limitation, as well as all obstructive airway apneas. It records but does not attempt to treat an apnea if the airway is open (i.e., central apnea). After responding to an airway problem, the device gradually reduces pressure until the next event restricting airflow. {{COLSPAN}} *AutoSet Clinical* is for professional attended use with an external dosimeter to gather information on respiratory parameters and oxygen saturation. In *autosetting mode*, it monitors and treats a patient during sleep and can recommend a treatment pressure for a standard CPAP device (replacing the traditional titration study). In *manual mode* it delivers a predetermined CPAP pressure. {{COLSPAN}} *AutoSet Portable II* is for unattended use by a professional and operates in all modes. {{COLSPAN}} The *AutoSet T* is a new device, not yet marketed, for long term treatment at home. It is capable of continually varying the treatment pressure automatically, based on the ongoing analysis of patient events and response *(autosetting mode)*. *AutoSet T* is awaiting FDA clearance. Studies of efficacy have been presented in professional meetings and peer-reviewed journals. **For masks, see ResMed Sullivan V listing.**				
Respironics Virtuoso™LX Smart CPAP System	The Virtuoso Smart CPAP devices are designed around the premise that complete (apnea) or partial (hypopnea) airway collapse is preceded by airway instability and vibration. A pressure transducer and a microprocessor are used to monitor the airway for vibration patterns that typically preceed airway collapse. When instability is detected, presure is increased, and when instability is absent, pressure is reduced. Peak pressures are similar to those established under manual titration, but pressure is adjusted to changing patient response. While the system does not abolish all apneas or hypopneas, it is claimed to reduce the apnea/hypopnea index (AHI) to acceptable levels. Clinical studies demonstrated that the Virtuoso System reduced AHI to below 10 at a lower average airway pressure compared to manual titration, however manually titrated CPAP achieved a greater improvement in AHI. Studies of efficacy have been presented in professional meetings and peer-reviewed journals. System can provide CPAP, Auto-CPAP, and split night with Auto-CPAP. {{COLSPAN}} The device weighs 3.5lb (1.6 kg.) and can accept 115 VAC or 230VAC and 12VDC. Other features include storage of daily usage records and therapy levels. Automatic pressure on/off feature, compensates for elevation changes and most leaks, optional alarm if mask is removed. **For masks, see Respironics Solo listing.**				
Sunrise/DeVilbiss Horizon™ AutoAdjust™ CPAP System, AutoAdjust™LT	Horizon AutoAdjust CPAP automatically adjusts pressure throughout the night based on patient need. Internal pressure and flow sensors monitor the patient on a breath-by-breath basis, looking for abnormal flow patterns caused by obstructive apnea, hypopnea, and snoring. Based on analysis of series of these abnormal flow patterns, pressure is gradually raised until the abnormal flow is eliminated, then the pressure is gradually reduced. By responding to the changing pressure needs, average airway pressure can be reduced while meeting peak needs. This device is designed to treat variable pressure requirements during each night as well as night-to-night differences. Patients who cannot tolerate standard CPAP may find the AutoAdjust more comfortable. Studies of efficacy have been presented in professional meetings and peer-reviewed journals. {{COLSPAN}} In combination with the separate Surveyor™ monitor device, the AutoAdjust can be used by clinicians to assess the patient's need for pressure and can record an eight-hour respiratory-event study with six separate data channels.The AutoAdjust and Surveyor combination can be used by clinicians to perform automatic CPAP titration in the sleep lab or home, thus reducing the delay between diagnosis and titration and treatment. {{COLSPAN}} Other features include storage of daily usage records, and initiation and cessation of CPAP flow in response to patient breathing. Specifications for filter, size and weight, and electrical are like the Horizon STandard. {{COLSPAN}} AutoAdjustLT, soon to be released, will have configuration similar to the Horizon LT CPAP device, technical specifications not available at this time. **For masks, see ResMed Sunrise/DeVilbiss Horizon LT listing.**				

a. This information is based on product sheets, web sites, and promotional literature provided by the manufacturer of each device and the claims have not been evaluated. Inclusion in this list does not imply endorsement, nor does omission imply a negative evaluation. Due to a number of acquisitions and mergers in this industry, and the rapid pace of research and development, specific models listed here may not be available and the names and features of currently available models may differ from those reported here. Specific devices and masks depicted in *Table D.2, Illustrations of CPAPP devices and masks*, may not be current models or names. Readers seeking the latest information may visit the Phantom Sleep Resources Page <http://www.newtechpub.com/phantom> or the web pages of the several manufacturers which are listed in Appendix A and on the Phantom Sleep Resources Page. This revision: June, 1998.

Table D.2   Illustrations of CPAP devices and masks[a]

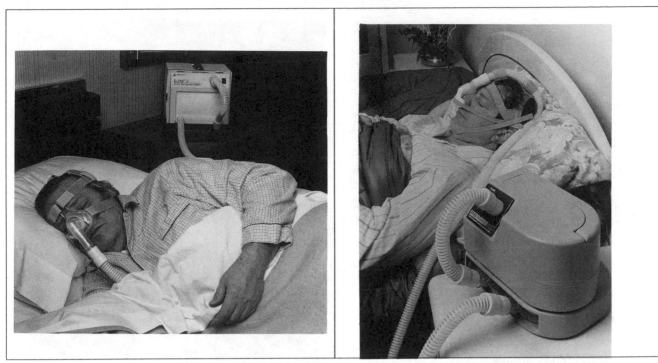

Left   A patient using the BiPAP S Airway Management System with humidifier; note the hose runs under the blanket, apparently to warm the air.

Right   ADAM circuit and Companion 318 by Nellcor Puritan Bennett. An improved model of the ADAM circuit shown is available. See next page for Companion 318 Plus.

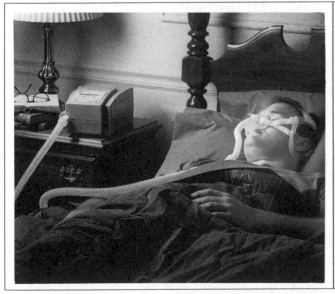 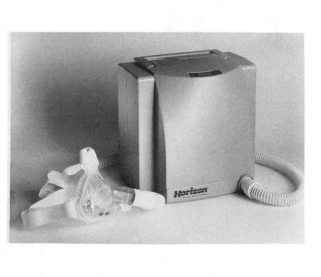

Left   Aria CPAP System by Respironics with Monarch Mini Mask which fits under the nose.

Right   Horizon nasal CPAP by DeVilbiss. The Horizon AutoAdjust CPAP is similar in appearance.

Table D.2   Illustrations of CPAP devices and masks[a]

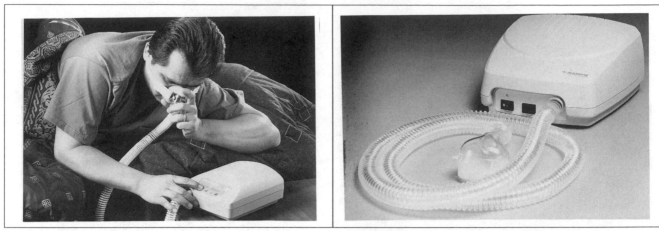

Left	The Lifecare CPAP-200 shown in use.
Right	Tranquility Quest nasal CPAP system by Healthdyne Technologies

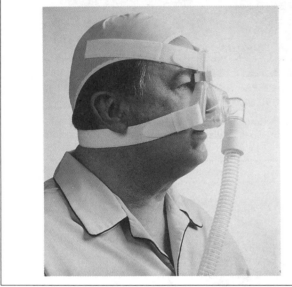

Left	Wearing a nasal mask using the Softcap by Respironics.
Right	Sullivan Bubble Cushion by ResMed.

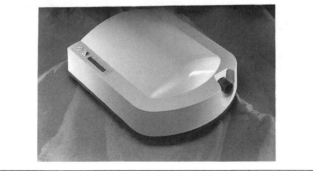
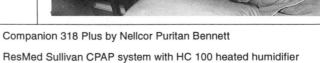

Left	Companion 318 Plus by Nellcor Puritan Bennett
Right	ResMed Sullivan CPAP system with HC 100 heated humidifier

Table D.2   Illustrations of CPAP devices and masks[a]

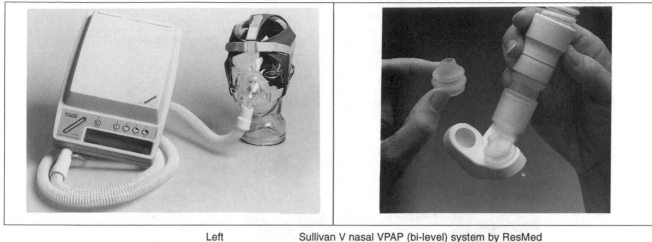

Left	Sullivan V nasal VPAP (bi-level) system by ResMed
Right	Detail of ADAM circuit showing inserting puffs

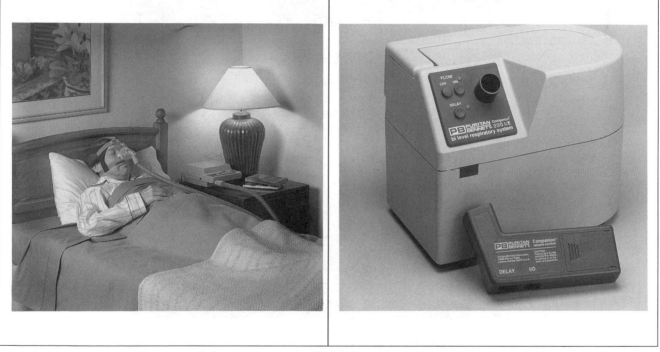

Left   ResMed Sullivan V CPAP system with Sullivan® mask, and ResCap headgear.

Right   Nellcor Puritan Bennett Companion® 320 I/E bi-level respiratory system and remote control.

a. This information is based on illustrations provided by the manufacturer of each device. Inclusion does not imply endorsement, nor does exclusion imply a negative evaluation.

Table D.3   Home monitoring systems[a]

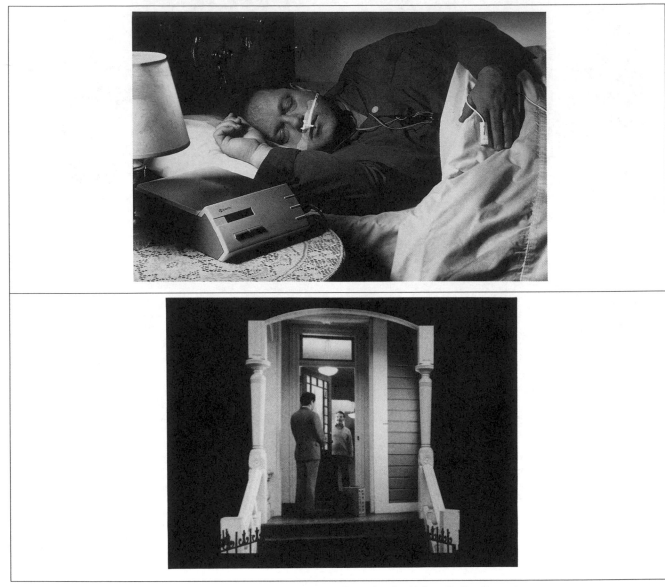

Unattended overnight recording using the Nellcor Puritan Bennet EdenTrace system.

A technician arrives to set up a patient for an overnight study, bringing a VISTA Polysomnography System by TeleDiagnostic Systems.

a. This table is based on information and illustrations provided by the manufacturer of each device. Inclusion does not imply endorsement, nor does omission imply a negative evaluation.

Glossary

active sleep—another term for dream (REM) sleep.

alpha waves—brain waves that occur eight to twelve times per second; these waves are most evident when a person is relaxed with eyes closed but not asleep.

apnea index—(AI) the number of apneas observed in an hour of sleep

apnea plus hypopnea index—(AHI) the number of apneas and hypopneas in an hour of sleep

apnea—"without breath," an interruption in the normal flow of air in and out of the body.

arousal—a brief awakening, complete or partial, from sleep.

arrhythmia—irregular rhythm of the heart

automatic behavior—performing routine tasks, such as driving a car, while in a daze, with partial or complete amnesia after the activity.

AWAKE—A mutual help group for persons with sleep-disordered breathing and their families.

beta waves—brain waves that occur more than thirteen times per second.

bi-level positive airway pressure—(BiPAP) a more complex form of CPAP that provides two different levels of pressure, higher during inhalation and lower during exhalation.

calibration—the confirmation that instruments are measuring correctly by using a known standard.

cannulae, nasal—tubes that fit slightly inside the nose to provide for delivery of CPAP

cataplexy—brief episodes of sudden muscle weakness usually brought on by surprise or emotion (laughter, anger). A characteristic symptom of narcolepsy.

central (sleep) apnea—interruption in breathing during sleep due to failure of activation of the muscles of breathing.

circadian—biological processes or events that occur on a daily schedule.

cm—abbreviation for centimeter, a metric unit of length; there are 2.54 centimeters to an inch.

CPAP—Continuous Positive Airway Pressure; a machine that delivers air under pressure for the treatment of sleep apnea.

delta sleep—deep non-REM sleep during which the majority of brain waves are delta waves.

delta waves—brain waves that occur from zero to four times per second.

depression—an alteration in mood having many symptoms similar to sleep apnea, such as feeling down or lethargic, lacking interest in social events, having no energy, trouble concentrating, poor memory, sense of failure in relationships.

desaturation—a lowering of the level of blood oxygen so that it is less saturated with oxygen. Marks a sleep apnea.

diaphragm—the main muscle of breathing, which lies between the chest and abdomen.

diving reflex—a slowing of the heart rate seen when diving mammals (seals, porpoises) hold their breath and dive underwater. A similar reflex may slow the heart beat in patients experiencing apnea.

dream sleep—REM sleep.

EDS—excessive daytime sleepiness.

EEG—electroencephalogram—the recording produced by measuring brain waves.

EMG—electromyogram—the recording produced by measuring muscle tension, usually on the chin.

EOG—electrooculogram—the recording produced by electrodes measuring eye movements.

excessive daytime sleepiness—(EDS) tendency to fall asleep in the daytime, a cardinal symptom of sleep apnea, narcolepsy, and other sleep disorders.

hyoid bone—a horseshoe-shaped bone in the neck attached to some of the muscles of the throat.

hypopnea—partial obstructive apnea in which airflow continues but at a much reduced level; usually associated with oxygen desaturation.

insomnia—the inability to fall asleep or stay asleep.

K complexes—an EEG feature typical of stage 2 sleep

lower airway—air passages from the voice box down the windpipe and into the lung.

mandible—the lower jaw.

manometer—a device that measures pressure.

maxilla—the upper jaw.

micro-arousal—partial awakening from sleep of which the sleeper is unaware.

micro-sleep—a brief sleep episode that intrudes into waking, typically experienced by sleep-deprived persons.

mixed (sleep) apnea—interruption in breathing during sleep which begins as a central apnea then becomes an obstructive apnea.

MSLT—multiple sleep latency test.

Multiple sleep latency test—daytime test done in a sleep laboratory to determine if the patient is excessively sleepy; consists of a series of naps during the day with measurement of the brain waves. Measures how long it takes to fall asleep compared to a set of norms.

narcolepsy—a disease of daytime sleep attacks, disturbed nighttime sleep, and, in many patients, cataplexy; other symptoms include sleep paralysis and sleep-related hallucinations.

nasal cannulae, nasal puffs, nasal seal—see cannulae, nasal.

nasal septum—the tissue that separates the left and right half of the nose; a deviated nasal septum may obstruct the nasal passages and cause sleep apnea.

nasal turbinates—fleshy outgrowths of tissue in the nasal cavity that warm and humidify air as it enters the body.

nocturia—the need for frequent urination during the night; may be a symptom of sleep apnea.

nocturnal myoclonus—a condition in which frequent jerks of the limbs disturb sleep.

non-REM sleep—quiet sleep, slow-wave sleep; about 80 percent of sleep; characterized by slower and larger brain waves and little or no dream behavior.

occlusion—the nasal mask seals off the skin from exposure to the air, thus the skin can become damp and possibly irritated.

obstructive (sleep) apnea—interruption of breathing during sleep due to a blockage of airflow through the upper airway.

paradoxical sleep—another term for dream or REM sleep.

pharynx—throat and accompanying structures.

polygraph—recording machine used in a sleep study; produces a polygram or polysomnogram.

positive pressure therapy—the use of air pressure applied through a nasal or face mask to eliminate apneas; devices include CPAP and BiPAP.

prongs—another term for cannulae, nasal.

PSG—polysomnogram—the recording of many types of information about a sleeping person that is made in a sleep laboratory.

pulmonologist—a specialist in breathing and diseases of the lung.

quiet sleep—non-REM sleep.

rebound effect—increase in the amount of certain types of sleep seen after sleep deprivation or the discontinuation of sleeping pills.

REM sleep, rapid eye movement sleep—sleep characterized by active brain waves, flitting motions of the eyes, and weakness of the muscles; most dreaming occurs in this stage, which accounts for about 20% of sleep in adults.

resolution—as in resolution of snoring, means the elimination of snoring by a treatment.

rhinitis—irritation or inflammation of the nasal passages.

risk factor—a person is at greater risk for a disease if they have the risk factor.

SAS—sleep apnea syndrome.

sign—objective evidence (such as a fast heart beat) that suggests that a disease is present.

sleep apnea syndrome—symptoms (complaints by patients, such as excessive daytime sleepiness or EDS) and signs (physical clues to disease observed by physicians, such as a narrow throat) that result from or may identify causes of interrupted breathing during sleep.

sleep apnea—interruption in breathing during sleep.

sleep efficiency—the percentage of time in bed which is spent in sleep; usually exceeds ninety percent in normal subjects studied in a sleep laboratory.

sleep hygiene—efforts to improve sleep by modifying habits and behaviors.

sleep latency—the time required to fall asleep once lights are turned out.

sleep spindles—brief bursts of fast brain waves that indicate sleep; primarily seen in stage 2 sleep.

soft palate—the soft, movable part of the roof of the mouth.

stoma—an opening into the body, usually surgically created.

supine—lying flat on one's back.

symptom—subjective complaints or observations that a patient relates to a doctor.

syndrome—a constellation of symptoms and signs of disease that often occur together but which may be caused by many disease processes.

theta waves—brain waves that occur four to seven times per second.

titration—the progressive, stepwise increase in CPAP pressure applied during a polysomnogram to establish the optimal treatment pressure.

tracheostomy—operation to create a breathing hole in the windpipe (trachea).

upper airway—the structures that air flows through on its way to the windpipe and lungs, consisting of nose and mouth passages and the throat; used for swallowing, speech, and breathing.

uvula—almond-size appendage hanging down in back of throat.

uvulopalatopharyngoplasty—operation performed on the throat to treat snoring and sleep apnea; abbreviated as UPPP, UPP, or UP3.

Bibliography

Snoring and sleep apnea

Ferber, Richard, *Solve Your Child's Sleep Problems*, New York: Simon and Schuster, 1985.

Lipman, Derek S., M.D., *Stop Your Husband from Snoring: A medically proven program to cure the night's worst nuisance.* Emmaus, Penn.: Rodale Press, 1990.

Lipman, Derek S., M.D., *Snoring from A to ZZZZZ: Proven Cures for the Night's Worst Nuisance*, 1996

Mosley, James L., *Snore No More! How to help your mate or family member stop snoring and live longer. Modern technology and information makes it possible.* Cleveland: 1996

Pascualy, Ralph A. M.D., and Sally Warren Soest, *Snoring and Sleep Apnea: Personal and Family Guide to Diagnosis and Treatment*, New York: Raven Press, 1994; New York: Demos Vermande, 1996

Sleep and sleep disorders

Borbély, Alexander, *Secrets of Sleep*, New York: Basic Books, 1986.

Dement, William Charles, *The Sleepwatchers*, Stanford: Stanford Alumni Association, 1992.

Dement, William Charles, *Some Must Watch While Some Must Sleep*, Stanford: Stanford Alumni Association, 1976.

Coleman, Richard M., *Wide Awake at 3:00 A.M., By Choice or by Chance?*, New York: W.H. Freeman and Company, 1986.

Ferber, Richard, *Solve Your Child's Sleep Problems*, New York: Simon and Schuster, 1985.

Fritz, Roger, *Sleep Disorders: America's Hidden Nightmare*, Naperville, IL: National Sleep Alert, Inc., 1993.

Hauri, Peter, Ph.D. and Shirley Linde, Ph.D.; *No More Sleepless Nights*, New York: John Wiley & Sons, Inc., 1990.

Hobson, J. Allan, *The Dreaming Brain*, New York: Basic Books, 1988.

Hobson, J. Allan, *Sleep*, New York: W. H. Freeman & Co., 1989.

Horne, James, *Why We Sleep: the Functions of Sleep in Humans and Other Mammals*, New York: Oxford University Press, 1988

Lamberg, Lynne, *The American Medical Association Guide to Better Sleep*, New York: Random House, 1984

Moore-Ede, Martin, *The Twenty Four Hour Society: Understanding Human Limits in a World That Never Stops*, Reading, MA: Addison-Wesley, 1993.

National Commission on Sleep Disorders Research, *Wake Up America: A National Sleep Alert—Report of the National Commission on Sleep Disorders Research*, Department of Health and Human Services Pub. No. 92-xxxx; Washington, D.C.: Superintendent of Documents, U.S. Government Printing Office, 1992

Regestein, Q.R., David Ritchie, and the editors of Consumer Reports Books, *Sleep: Problems and Solutions*, Mount Vernon, New York: Consumers Union, 1990.

Regestein, Quentin R., M.D., with J. R. Rechs, *Sound Sleep*, New York: Simon & Schuster, 1980.

U.S. Department of Health and Human Services, Public Health Service, National Institutes of Health, *Breathing Disorders During Sleep*, NIH Publication No. 93-2966

Sleep and sleep disorders—professional literature

AHCPR (Agency for Health Care Policy and Research), Polysomnography and Sleep Disorder Centers, Health Technology Assessment Reports, 1991, Number 4, U.S. Department of Health and Human Services, Public Health Service, Agency for Health Care Policy and Research, Rockville, Maryland; May, 1992, AHCPR Publication 92-0027

Guilleminault, Christian (ed.), *Sleeping and waking disorders: indications and techniques*. Boston: Butterworths, 1982

Hobson, J.A., and M. Steriade, "Neuronal basis of behavioral state control," pp. 701-823 in: V. Mountcastle and F. E. Bloom, eds., *Handbook of Physiology: The Nervous System, Vol. IV*, Bethesda, Maryland: American Physiological Association, 1986

Kryger, Meir, T. Roth, and W. C. Dement, *The Principles and Practices of Sleep Medicine*, Philadelphia: W.B. Saunders Co., 1989

Kryger, Meir, M.D., editor, with Mark Sanders, MD, John Shepard, MD, Jim Walsh, Ph.D., Philip Westbrook, MD: *Sleep Apnea: Physiology and Diagnosis*, Slide Series; *sixty slides and text for health professionals*, published by the American Sleep Disorders Association

Standards of Practice Committee of the American Sleep Disorders Association, "Practice Parameters for the Treatment of Obstructive Sleep Apnea in Adults: The Efficacy of Surgical Modifications of the Upper Airway," *Sleep*, 19(2): 152-155, 1996

Standards of Practice Committee of the American Sleep Disorders Association, "Practice Parameters for the Treatment of Snoring and Obstructive Sleep Apnea with Oral Appliances," *Sleep*, 18(6): 511-513, 1995

Thorpy, M. J., Chairman, Diagnostic Classification Steering Committee, *International classification of sleep disorders: Diagnostic and coding manual*, Rochester: American Sleep Disorders Association, 1990

Related health topics

Sacks, Oliver, *Awakenings*, New York: Harper/Collins, 1990

Sataloff, Robert T., "The Human Voice," *Scientific American*, Volume 267, Number 6, December, 1992, pp. 108-115.

Winson, Jonathan, 1990, "The Meaning of Dreams" *Scientific American*, November 1990, pp. 86-96.

The health care system

Callahan, Daniel, *What Kind of Life: The Limits of Medical Progress*, New York: Touchstone/Simon & Schuster, Inc. 1990

Life style, nutrition, and weight loss

Ornish, Dean, M.D., *Dr. Dean Ornish's Program for Reversing Heart Disease*, New York: Ballantine 1990

Periodicals, articles, pamphlets, slides

American Sleep Apnea Association, *APNEWS;* A quarterly newsletter for people who have sleep apnea.

American Sleep Disorders Association, *Don't Take Sleep Problems Lying Down.*

American Sleep Disorders Association, *Insomnia.*

American Sleep Disorders Association, *Sleep as We Grow Older.*

American Sleep Disorders Association, *Sleep Disorders Centers: What are they? What do they do?*

American Sleep Disorders Association, *Sleep Problems in Children: A Parent's Guide.*

AWAKE Network (American Sleep Apnea Association), *The AWAKE Network;* A newsletter for coordinators of AWAKE health awareness groups for individuals with sleep disordered breathing.

AWAKE Network (American Sleep Apnea Association), *AWAKE Organizational Guidelines*, Seger, Lucy, Nancy Kern, and Joyce Black; *A guide to starting and organizing a new group.*

Baird, William P., *Narcolepsy: A nonmedical presentation*, The American Narcolepsy Association, Inc., 1987.

Baird, William P., *Sleep Apnea: A non-technical presentation*, The American Narcolepsy Association, Inc., 1977, 1988.

Blitzer, Bud, editor, International Ventilator Users Network. (I.V.U.N.) *Directory of Sources for Ventilation Face Masks*, St. Louis: Gazette International Networking Institute. *Photographs and descriptions of custom and ready-to-use face masks for CPAP, also intermittent positive pressure ventilation masks that can also be used for CPAP, with price, laboratories, and manufacturer listings.*

I.V.U.N. News, Spring and Fall, St. Louis: Gazette International Networking Institute.

Lamberg, Lynne, *Sleep Apnea: Symptoms, causes, evaluation, treatment;* American Sleep Disorders Association. 1987.

Sleep/Wake Disorders organization, *Keeping Awake*, newsletter of the Sleep/Wake Disorders organization, Canada.

Internet & Web information sources

New Technology Publishing, Inc., maintains *Phantom sleep resources (apnea, snoring and other sleep concerns)* <**http://www.newtechpub.com**> on the World Wide Web, a source of information and news in sleep apnea and snoring. It covers developments including research, treatment, and support, as well as products and services and contains a guide, "Sleeping on the Net," with links to internet sites, resources, and news groups. Submissions, comments, and queries to Jerry Halberstadt at <*jerry@newtechpub.com*>.

Index

About the authors and contributors

T. Scott Johnson, M.D.

T. Scott Johnson, M.D., a pulmonologist and expert in sleep disorders, has been the Director of the Sleep Disorders Center, USA-Knollwood Park Hospital, and associate professor of medicine at the University of South Alabama College of Medicine, Mobile, Alabama. He has also been the medical director of the Sleep Laboratory at Beth Israel Hospital, Boston, Massachusetts and the Sleep Disorders Service at Brigham and Women's Hospital, Boston, and assistant professor of medicine at Harvard University Medical School. He has engaged in research to develop methods for identifying, diagnosing, and treating sleep apnea syndrome patients and has overseen the establishment of a sleep laboratory at a hospital in Hamburg, Germany.

Jerry Halberstadt

Jerome (Jerry) Halberstadt has suffered from SAS for more than 15 years. His frustrations in obtaining appropriate treatment in both Israel and the United States led him to seek information to help him take a more active, effective role in his treatment and rehabilitation. As an anthropologist, he has studied Navaho community curing rituals and has worked in planning educational, medical, mental health, and community development activities and services in the United States and in Israel. He is a publisher and book developer as well as a consumer of health care services.

William Charles Dement

William Charles Dement, M.D., Ph.D. is Professor of Psychiatry and Behavioral Sciences at the Stanford University School of Medicine. He has helped to found and lead the modern scientific study and treatment of sleep and wakefulness. In 1970 he founded the first Sleep Disorders Clinic, now the Stanford Sleep Disorders Clinic and Research Center and continues today as its director. He was appointed by the Secretary of Health and Human Services to serve as Chairman of the National Commission on Sleep Disorders Research, reporting to Congress with recommendations for a national sleep research program. He is recognized and esteemed by all researchers and clinicians in the field of sleep disorders. The committee that nominated Dr. Dement as the National

Institutes of Health Career Scientist wrote that he "...is an outstanding scientist of great energy, enthusiasm, and productivity, and who, more than any other individual, is responsible for the creation of a modern, viable field of sleep research, especially as it relates to sleep related pathologies."

Colin E. Sullivan

Dr. Colin E. Sullivan, B.Sc.(Med.), M.B. B.S., Ph.D., F.R.A.C.P. is the pioneer who invented and demonstrated nasal CPAP as an effective treatment for sleep apnea syndrome. The author of over 90 scientific publications, he has contributed signficantly to the development of sleep disorders medicine and his achievements are recognized internationally. In addition to his broad clinical and research interests, he has proved himself a creative inventor of devices for treating sleep apnea and is involved in their commercial development. Clearly motivated by a true physician's concern, Dr. Sullivan has a creative, forceful personality and his leadership qualities are backed by persistence; he has helped to transform sleep disorders medicine and the lives of multitudes of patients. He is Professor of Medicine, University of Sydney; Head, Sleep Disorders Centre, Royal Prince Alfred Hospital; and Head, David Read Pediatric Sleep Laboratory, Children's Hospital.

Boyd Hayes

Boyd Hayes consulted on sleep laboratory technical issues. He made and interpreted the sleep recordings used for base illustrations using the EdenTrace II and/or the Nicolet UltraSom computer systems for recording, analysis, and display, with confirming scorings by humans as appropriate. He also helped to research, write, and edit the manuscript. He is the Technical Director at Sleep Disorders Center, Dartmouth Hitchcock Medical Center, in Lebanon, NH. He has been Research Assistant at the Stanford Sleep Disorders Center and Sleep Technologist, Sleep Disorders Center, Dartmouth College, the Technical Director, Sleep Disorders Service, Brigham and Women's Hospital, Boston and a member of the ASDA Polysomnography Atlas Task Force.

Illustrations

Jim Roldan

Jim Roldan drew the sensitive illustrations opening each chapter, The three states of being: awake, quiet sleep, and dream sleep on page 14, and Out of touch on page 23, as well as the sleeping man in Figure 4.5 on page 38. He trained in illustration at the Rhode Island School of Design and his studio is in E. Hampstead, New Hampshire.

S. Kirsten Gay

The medical and technical illustrations were drawn by S. Kirsten Gay, an artist and illustrator with interests in garden design and architecture, who works at *Paradeisos Design,* Cambridge, MA. Ms. Gay trained in landscape architecture at Cornell University.

Editorial consultant

Marie Cantlon of *Proseworks,* Boston is the editor whose experience and sensitivity smoothed the completion of this work.

Design

David Margolin created the cover design and illustration and made helpful suggestions on the book design and illustrations, including the organization of Figure 4.5 on page 38.

Karyl Klopp made helpful suggestions on page layout.

Copyediting and Indexing

Mary Jane Curry and Wynter Snow read the manuscript during the development of the book; Lynne Gay assisted with the indexing.

Production

The text is set in Palatino with Helvetica heads, and the book was edited and output using FrameMaker software.

This book was printed and bound by BookCrafters.

Suggestions for future editions

How you can help us to help others

How can we make this book more useful? We are eager to receive your comments and additional experiences to so that others may be helped to overcome SAS. We welcome questions and suggestions as well as how you found this book helpful. Please point out any errors or omissions. We welcome patients' reports of experiences that demonstrate the spectrum of people who suffer from SAS, the range of problems created by untreated SAS, problems and triumphs in seeking diagnosis and treatment. We also seek the names and addresses of institutions, manufacturers, home care companies, patient education and support groups, and other resources which may be helpful.

Please write to New Technology Publishing and include your name and address so we will be able to follow up and clarify as needed, and so we can inform you of later editions and related publications. And please indicate where you learned about or obtained the book so we can learn how to make the book more readily available.

TO:
New Technology Publishing, Inc., Post Office Box 1737
Onset, Massachusetts, 02558-1737 USA
1-800-67-APNEA; email: newtech@newtechpub.com

Comments and suggestions from:

Name	
Street	
City	
State, Zip	
Telephone	
I obtained or learned about this book from :	
This book should be available at:	

Please use as many pages as necessary; copy this page as needed.

Questionnaire for a friend

Questions to Identify sleep apnea syndrome

✄ Answering the questions below will help you to understand whether sleep apnea is disturbing your sleep and disrupting your life. The questions marked ♠ are especially important; a "yes" answer strongly suggests that sleep apnea is the problem. To answer questions marked with a ♥, you will need the help of your roommate, bedmate, or a family member, or you may use a tape recorder to identify snoring and pauses in breathing. For information on how to use a tape recorder for this purpose, see *Phantom of the Night*.

During sleep and in the bedroom

❑ *Do you snore loudly each night?* ♠♥

❑ *Do you have frequent pauses in breathing while you sleep (you stop breathing for ten seconds or longer)?* ♠♥

❑ Are you restless during sleep, tossing and turning from one side to another?♥

❑ Does your posture during sleep seem unusual—do you sleep sitting up or propped up by pillows?♥

❑ Do you have insomnia–waking up frequently and without a reason?

❑ Do you have to get up to urinate several times during the night?

❑ Have you wet your bed?

❑ Have you fallen from bed?

While awake

❑ Do you wake up in the morning tired and foggy, not ready to face the day?

❑ Do you have headaches in the morning? ♠

❑ Are you very sleepy during the day? ♠

❑ Do you fall asleep easily during the day? ♠

❑ Do you have difficulty concentrating, being productive, and completing tasks at work?

❑ Do you carry out routine tasks in a daze?

❑ Have you ever arrived home in your car but couldn't remember the trip from work?

Adjustment and emotional issues

☐ Are you having serious relationship problems at home, with friends and relatives, or at work?

☐ Are you afraid that you may be out of touch with the real world, unable to think clearly, losing your memory, or emotionally ill?

☐ Do your friends tell you that you're not like yourself?

☐ Are you depressed?

☐ Are you irritable and angry, especially first thing in the morning?

Medical, physical condition, and lifestyle

☐ Are you overweight?

☐ Do you have high blood pressure?

☐ Do you have pains in your bones and joints?

☐ Do you have trouble breathing through your nose?

☐ Do you often have a drink of alcohol before going to bed?

☐ If you are a man, is your collar size 17 inches (42 centimeters) or larger?

What your answers may mean

A "yes" answer to *any* of these questions may be a clue that an underlying disease exists. That disease may be sleep apnea, another sleep disorder, or a problem not related to sleep. Each of the questions points to a symptom. Symptoms are the clues, sometimes subtle and perceived only by the patient (such as memory loss), and sometimes overt and observable by friend or family (such as snoring) that indicate that the mind or body is diseased. Your doctor, trained to see symptoms as the manifestation of disease, can help you interpret and understand the basis of your condition. For more information to help in diagnosis, treatment, and recovery, read *Phantom of the Night.*

To order *Phantom of the Night*, ISBN 1-882431-02-2, $29.95, at the *prepaid* price of $26.95, enclose payment with this form to New Technology Publishing, Inc., Post Office Box 1737, Onset, Massachusetts, 02558-1737 USA
To order at the list price of $29.95: Please submit your name, address, phone, fax, and email to us at
Telephone: 1-800-67-APNEA Electronic mail on Internet: <newtech@newtechpub.com>

	Price	Number	Total		Sold to/ship to
Each copy, 1-4 books *prepaid*	$26.95			Name	
Each copy, 1-4 books	$29.95			Name	
Mass. residents 5% tax				Address	
Additional international shipping				City	
TOTAL			$	State, Zip, Country	
				Telephone	

To save time, order by phone or electronic mail at the list price of $29.95. The Mass. tax of 5% on $29.95 is $1.50, on $26.95 is $1.35. Priority Mail shipping is included on orders for up to 10 books in the U.S.
INTERNATIONAL ORDERS: For faster, more economical service: please order through your local patient support organization—they may have copies in stock. Payable in US dollars drawn on a bank branch located in the United States or by International Postal Money Order. Air: Canada & Mexico, $3.95; other Western Hemisphere, $5.95; W. Europe, $3.95; Asia & Africa, $8.68; Pacific Rim, $6.95. *For larger quantities, price, shipping and insurance will be quoted.*

Order forms

Prepaid orders

To order *Phantom of the Night*, ISBN 1-882431-02-2, $29.95
at the *prepaid* price of $26.95, please enclose payment with a copy of this form to New Technology Publishing, Inc.,
Post Office Box 1737, Onset, Massachusetts, 02558-1737 USA

	Price	Quantity	Total
Each copy, 1-4 books *prepaid*	$26.95		
Each copy, 5-10 books *prepaid*	$23.95		
Each copy, in case lot of 30, *prepaid to patient support group members* Please call for best discount.	Call for lowest price		
Massachusetts residents please add 5% tax			
Additional shipping per book outside USA (see International orders below)			
Shipping & Handling on case lots in USA per case	$35.00		
			$

Priority Mail shipping is included on orders for up to 10 books in the U.S. For faster service, order by phone or electronic mail at the list price of $29.95: 1-800-67-APNEA, email: <newtech@newtechpub.com> or <http://www.newtechpub.com>
INTERNATIONAL ORDERS FOR SINGLE COPIES: Payable in advance with US dollars drawn on a bank branch located in the United States or by International Postal Money Order. Additional Air Mail Postage outside USA: Canada & Mexico, $3.95; other Western Hemisphere, $5.95; Western Europe (Austria, Belgium, Denmark, Finland, France, Germany, Great Britain, Iceland, Ireland, Luxembourg, Netherlands, Norway, Portugal, Spain, Sweden, Switzerland), $3.95, other Europe, $8.95; Asia & Africa, $8.68; Pacific Rim (Australia, Hong Kong, Japan, New Zealand, Philipines, Singapore, S. Korea, Taiwan, Thailand, Vietnam),$5.95, other Pacific rim $12.13. *For larger quantities, price, shipping and insurance will be quoted.* Please contact your nearest patient support group (see partial list under Organizations on page 121), several stock and distribute the book or they can arrange a group purchase.

SOLD TO:	SHIP TO:
Name	Name
Title	Title
Department	Department
Company	Company
Street	Street
City	City
State, Zip	State, Zip
Telephone	Telephone
FAX	FAX

Order form for corporate and institutional accounts

Order *Phantom of the Night*, ISBN 1-882431-02-2, $29.95 from
New Technology Publishing, Inc.,
Post Office Box 9183, Cambridge, Massachusetts, 02139-9183 USA
Telephone: 508-291-1111 or 617-661-3851; 1-800-67-APNEA; FAX: 1-800-45-APNEA; 508-291-1704
Electronic mail on Internet: <halberst@world.std.com> Visit our site at <http://newtechpub.com>

Quantity and terms	Price	Quantity	Total
Each copy, 1-10 books, net 30 (Priority Mail in US included)	$29.95		
Each copy, 11-30 books, net 30	$23.95		
Each copy, 30 books (case lot), net 30	$17.97		
Each copy, 1-4 books, *prepaid* (Priority Mail in US included)	$26.95		
Each copy, 5-10 books, *prepaid* (Priority Mail in US included)	$23.95		
Massachusetts purchasers add 5% tax (or exempt certificate)			
Shipping on 11 or more books in USA			
Shipping outside USA			
			$

CORPORATE and INSTITUTIONAL orders with purchase order number can be placed by phone, FAX , mail, or electronic mail. Terms:2% 10/ Net 30 days. Ground freight and insurance will be billed on orders for 11 or more books. Call for quotes on larger quantities.

INTERNATIONAL ORDERS: Payable in US dollars drawn on a bank branch located in the United States or by International Postal Money Order. Additional Air Mail Postage outside USA: Canada, $3.95; Mexico, $2.20; other Western Hemisphere, $3.75; Western Europe (Austria, Belgium, Denmark, Finland, France, Germany, Great Britain, Iceland, Ireland, Luxembourg, Netherlands, Norway, Portugal, Spain, Sweden, Switzerland), $6.60, other Europe, $8.95; Asia & Africa, $8.68; Pacific Rim (Australia, Hong Kong, Japan, New Zealand, Philipines, Singapore, S. Korea, Taiwan, Thailand, Vietnam),$5.95, other Pacific rim $12.13. *For larger quantities, price, shipping and insurance will be quoted.* Please contact your nearest patient support group (see partial list under Organizations on page 121), several stock and distribute the book or they can arrange a group purchase.

SOLD TO (reader/department ordering):	SHIP TO:
Name	Name
Title	Title
Department	Department
Company	Company
Street	Street
City	City
State, Zip, Country	State, Zip, Country
Telephone	Telephone

PURCHASE ORDER NUMBER

SIGNATURE

DATE

Name

Title

Telephone

FAX